ORTHOPEDIC CLINICS OF NORTH AMERICA

www.orthopedic.theclinics.com

Soft Tissue Procedures

July 2022 • Volume 53 • Number 3

Editor-in-Chief
FREDERICK M. AZAR

Editorial Board
MICHAEL J. BEEBE
CLAYTON C. BETTIN
TYLER J. BROLIN
JAMES H. CALANDRUCCIO
CHRISTOPHER T. COSGROVE
BENJAMIN J. GREAR
BENJAMIN M. MAUCK
WILLIAM M. MIHALKO
BENJAMIN SHEFFER
KIRK M. THOMPSON
PATRICK C. TOY

ELSEVIER

1600 John F. Kennedy Boulevard • Suite 1800 • Philadelphia, Pennsylvania, 19103-2899.

http://www.orthopedic.theclinics.com

ORTHOPEDIC CLINICS OF NORTH AMERICA Volume 53, Number 3
July 2022 ISSN 0030-5898, ISBN-13: 978-0-323-98763-9

Editor: Megan Ashdown
Developmental Editor: Ann Gielou Posedio

Orthopedic Clinics of North America (ISSN 0030-5898) is published quarterly by Elsevier Inc., 360 Park Avenue South, New York, NY 10010-1710. Months of issue are January, April, July, and October. Business and Editorial Offices: 1600 John F. Kennedy Blvd., Suite 1800, Philadelphia, PA 19103-2899. Customer Service Office: 3251 Riverport Lane, Maryland Heights, MO 63043. Periodicals postage paid at New York, NY and additional mailing offices. Subscription prices are $354.00 per year for (US individuals), $1,033.00 per year for (US institutions), $420.00 per year (Canadian individuals), $1,064.00 per year (Canadian institutions), $486.00 per year (international individuals), $1,064.00 per year (international institutions), $100.00 per year (US students), $100.00 per year for (Canadian students), $220.00 per year for (international students). Foreign air speed delivery is included in all *Clinics* subscription prices. All prices are subject to change without notice. **POSTMASTER:** Send change of address to *Orthopedic Clinics of North America*, **Elsevier Health Sciences Division, Subscription Customer Service, 3251 Riverport Lane, Maryland Heights, MO 63043. Customer Service (orders, claims, online, change of address): Elsevier Health Sciences Division, Subscription Customer Service, 3251 Riverport Lane, Maryland Heights, MO 63043. Tel: 1-800-654-2452 (U.S. and Canada); 314-447-8871 (outside U.S. and Canada). Fax: 314-447-8029. E-mail:** journalscustomerservice-usa@elsevier.com **(for print support);** journalsonlinesupport-usa@elsevier.com **(for online support).**

Reprints. For copies of 100 or more, of articles in this publication, please contact the Commercial Reprints Department, Elsevier Inc., 360 Park Avenue South, New York, NY 10010-1710. Tel.: 212-633-3874; Fax: 212-633-3820; E-mail: reprints@elsevier.com.

Orthopedic Clinics of North America is covered in *MEDLINE/PubMed* (*Index Medicus*), *Cinahl, Excerpta Medica*, and *Cumulative Index to Nursing and Allied Health Literature*.

EDITORIAL BOARD

CONTRIBUTORS

EDITOR

FREDERICK M. AZAR, MD
Chief of Staff, Campbell Clinic, Professor, Department of Orthopaedic Surgery and Biomedical Engineering, University of Tennessee/Campbell Clinic, Memphis, Tennessee, USA

AUTHORS

CHARLES LOWRY BARNES, MD
Department of Orthopaedic Surgery, University of Arkansas for Medical Sciences, Little Rock, Arkansas, USA

MICHAEL R. BISOGNO, MD, MBA
Orthopaedic Institute at Northwell Health, New York, New York, USA

JAMES A. BLAIR, MD, FACS
Associate Professor, Department of Orthopedic Surgery, Medical College of Georgia at Augusta University, Augusta, Georgia, USA

TYLER J. BROLIN, MD
Department of Orthopaedic Surgery and Biomedical Engineering, University of Tennessee-Campbell Clinic, Memphis, Tennessee, USA

JAMES CALANDRUCCIO, MD
Orthopaedic Surgeon, Associate Professor, Department of Orthopaedic Surgery and Biomedical Engineering, University of Tennessee Health Science Center - Campbell Clinic, Memphis, Tennessee, USA

JANA M. DAVIS, MD
Associate Professor, Department of Orthopedic Surgery, Medical College of Georgia at Augusta University, Augusta, Georgia, USA

THOMAS E. DICKERSON, BS
Medical Student, Medical College of Georgia at Augusta University, Augusta, Georgia, USA

HAYDEN D. FAITH, BS
Medical Student, Medical College of Georgia at Augusta University, Augusta, Georgia, USA

NOLAN FARRELL, MD
Orthopaedic Resident, Department of Orthopaedic Surgery and Biomedical Engineering, University of Tennessee Health Science Center - Campbell Clinic, Memphis, Tennessee, USA

JOHN GABRIEL HORNEFF III, MD
Assistant Professor of Clinical Orthopaedic Surgery, University of Pennsylvania, Philadelphia, Pennsylvania, USA

AARON JACOBS, MD
Division of Plastic and Reconstructive Surgery, Lehigh Valley Health Network, Allentown, Pennsylvania, USA

NICHOLAS JAMES, MD
Orthopedic Surgeon, Hand Fellow, Editorial Campbell Clinic Foundation, Memphis, Tennessee, USA

JAMES R. JASTIFER, MD
Clinical Associate Professor, Ascension Borgess Orthopedics, Western Michigan University Homer Stryker M.D. School of Medicine, Kalamazoo, Michigan, USA

FRANK G. LEE, BSE
University of South Florida Morsani College of Medicine, Allentown, Pennsylvania, USA

PETER A. LENNOX, MD, FRCS
Department of Surgery, Division of Plastic and Reconstructive Surgery, University of British Columbia, Vancouver, British Columbia, Canada

AHMED M. MANSOUR, MD
Division of Plastic and Reconstructive Surgery, Lehigh Valley Health Network, Allentown, Pennsylvania, USA

BASSAM A. MASRI, MD, FRCS
Department of Orthopaedics, University of
British Columbia, Vancouver, British
Columbia, Canada

BENJAMIN MAUCK, MD
Orthopaedic Surgeon, Assistant Professor,
Department of Orthopaedic Surgery and
Biomedical Engineering, University of
Tennessee Health Science Center - Campbell
Clinic, Memphis, Tennessee, USA

LYDIA J. MCKEITHAN, MD
Department of Orthopaedic Surgery,
University of California Davis, Sacramento,
California, USA

SIMON C. MEARS, MD, PhD
Department of Orthopaedic Surgery,
University of Arkansas for Medical Sciences,
Little Rock, Arkansas, USA

NATHAN F. MILLER, MD
Division of Plastic and Reconstructive Surgery,
Lehigh Valley Health Network, Allentown,
Pennsylvania, USA

ALEXA N. PEARCE, BA
Department of Orthopaedic Surgery,
University of Arkansas for Medical Sciences,
Little Rock, Arkansas, USA

WILLIAM POLIO, MD
Department of Orthopaedic Surgery and
Biomedical Engineering, University of
Tennessee-Campbell Clinic, Memphis,
Tennessee, USA

GEORGE A. PUNEKY, MD
Resident Physician, Department of
Orthopedic Surgery, Medical College of
Georgia at Augusta University, Augusta,
Georgia, USA

MAMTHA S. RAJ, MD, MA
Division of Plastic and Reconstructive Surgery,
Lehigh Valley Health Network, Allentown,
Pennsylvania, USA

BRANDON ANTHONY ROMERO, MD
Fellow, Shoulder and Elbow Division,
Department of Orthopaedics, University of
Pennsylvania, Philadelphia, Pennsylvania, USA

GILES R. SCUDERI, MD
Orthopaedic Institute at Northwell Health,
New York, New York, USA

GERARD A. SHERIDAN, MD, FRCS
Department of Orthopaedics, University of
British Columbia, Vancouver, British
Columbia, Canada

JEFFREY B. STAMBOUGH, MD
Department of Orthopaedic Surgery,
University of Arkansas for Medical Sciences,
Little Rock, Arkansas, USA

BENJAMIN M. STRONACH, MS, MD
Department of Orthopaedic Surgery,
University of Arkansas for Medical Sciences,
Little Rock, Arkansas, USA

WESTON TERRASSE, MD, MS
Division of Plastic and Reconstructive Surgery,
Lehigh Valley Health Network, Allentown,
Pennsylvania, USA

SEAN J. WALLACE, MD
Division of Plastic and Reconstructive Surgery,
Lehigh Valley Health Network, Easton,
Pennsylvania, USA

AMANDA T. WHITAKER, MD
Department of Orthopaedic Surgery, Shriners
Children's Hospital Northern California,
Assistant Professor of Orthopaedic Surgery,
Division of Pediatric Orthopaedics, University of
California Davis, Sacramento, California, USA

CONTENTS

Knee and Hip Reconstruction

Abductor insufficiency can cause abnormal gait, lateral hip pain, and abduction weakness in both native and prosthetic hips. In the setting of total hip arthroplasty (THA), abductor insufficiency may occur secondary to iatrogenic injury to the superior gluteal nerve or gluteus medius muscle, adverse local tissue reactions owing to metal-associated prosthetics, and osteolysis owing to bearing wear or infection. Surgical reconstruction of the abductor complex is indicated for patients with chronic tears who have pain, weakness, limp, and/or instability. This article reviews the pearls and pitfalls of surgical reconstruction options for abductor insufficiency following THA.

In the multiply operated on knee replacement, no one soft tissue procedure is vastly superior to another. The most extensive literature available is in relation to muscle flaps, which will continue to be the workhorse technique for orthopedic and plastic reconstructive surgeons for the foreseeable future. Closed incision negative pressure wound therapy may prove to be a superior method in time but further large-scale studies are required to expand our understanding of this technique. The continued use of a combination of these techniques, tailored to the specific patient, is likely to be the best approach to the multiply operated on knee into the future.

Extensor mechanism disruptions following total knee arthroplasty are devastating injuries with complication rates following surgical intervention ranging from 25% to 45%. Primary repair with and without augmentation is appropriate in certain limited clinical settings. Allograft reconstruction has been a popular option; however, synthetic grafts are showing promise and good results. In this article the authors discuss an algorithm for treating these difficult injuries as well as detail the surgical techniques for each approach.

Trauma

> Reconstruction plays a valuable role in the management of lower extremity
> wounds for limb salvage. The goals of reconstruction are to improve function
> and quality of life, return to work, and pain reduction while providing a long-
> lasting durable reconstruction. The plastics and reconstructive surgical
> approach in conjunction with the orthopedic or trauma team, referred often
> as the "orthoplastic" approach, can yield the best outcomes for patients.
> The following sections discuss reconstruction principles and techniques that
> can be applied broadly for lower extremity wounds secondary to trauma, infec-
> tion, and tumor resection.

> Soft tissue reconstructive techniques are powerful tools for the orthopedic sur-
> geon caring for lower extremity trauma. This article seeks to inform orthopedic
> surgeons about useful techniques for skin closure, secondary wound closure
> techniques, and rotational flaps of the lower leg. Split thickness skin grafting,
> piecrusting, and the use of negative pressure wound therapy for skin closure,
> as well as rotational gastrocnemius, soleus, and reverse sural artery flaps are
> discussed with emphasis on techniques for the nonvascular and nonmicrovas-
> cular orthopedic surgeon.

Pediatrics

> The transfer of the tibialis posterior tendon has been used to correct hindfoot
> varus and dorsiflexion weakness in cerebral palsy. It is expendable, has a favor-
> able direction for dorsiflexion and direction for dorsiflexion and eversion, and is
> the source of hindfoot varus in most cases. However, the foot and ankle must
> be flexible without skeletal deformity. The activity of the tibialis posterior
> should be present in the swing phase for the tendon transfer to function
> correctly as a dorsiflexor. Techniques and pitfalls are described to plan and
> execute a successful tibialis posterior tendon transfer.

Hand and Wrist

> The sagittal bands are structurally important, aiding in the central alignment of
> the extensor tendons over the heads of each metacarpal. They resist the devi-
> ation of the tendon with flexion of the metacarpophalangeal (MCP) joint. Injury
> to the sagittal band can cause the extensor tendon to lose its alignment lead-
> ing to pain, tendon subluxation, or dislocation. Generally, if these injuries are
> recognized and treated within 3 weeks of injury, they will not require surgery.
> The goal of surgery is to restore the anatomic alignment of the extensor
> tendon by either direct repair of the sagittal band or reconstruction.

Shoulder and Elbow

> Remplissage is a nonanatomic capsulotenodesis of the infraspinatus tendon used to fill engaging or "off-track" Hill-Sachs lesions in patients at high risk of recurrent instability with isolated Bankart repair. Indications for remplissage are expanding, as the importance of subcritical bone loss and the glenoid track on patient outcomes and recurrence rates continues to be investigated. Remplissage is also suggested in patients at high risk of recurrent instability following isolated anterior labral repair, such as collision and contact athletes with Hill-Sachs lesions that have not reached the threshold of "off track." Multiple arthroscopic remplissage techniques exist including, more recently, knotless techniques.

> Total shoulder arthroplasty is a rapidly growing field, with more procedures performed each year. An important aspect of shoulder arthroplasty surgery is the management of soft tissues. Good functional outcomes in shoulder arthroplasty are significantly dependent on the repair of the rotator cuff tendons and proper release of the shoulder capsule. The success of any shoulder arthroplasty is predicated upon the meticulous handling of these tissues. The surgeon's ability to execute appropriate soft tissue techniques will facilitate easier surgery by increasing exposure and lead to better outcomes for the patient.

Foot and Ankle

> The plantar plate is a known stabilizer of the lesser toe metatarsophalangeal (MTP) joint. MTP instability is a known common cause of metatarsalgia, most commonly in the second toe. In the last decade, clinical staging and anatomic grading mechanisms have been published to guide surgeons on the treatment of MTP instability; this has also led to an understanding of how plantar plate tears relate to MTP joint instability. Direct surgical repair of the plantar plate has been described, short-term outcomes have been published, and the results are not perfect, but promising with respect to patient satisfaction and pain relief.

SOFT TISSUE PROCEDURES

PREFACE

Damage to soft tissues often occurs during athletic activity or falls, with sprains, strains, contusions, and tendinitis being among the most common injuries. This issue reviews the latest surgical techniques and options available for repairing soft tissue damage so that good functional outcomes result.

Abductor insufficiency can cause abnormal gait, lateral hip pain, and abduction weakness in hips. When total hip arthroplasty is performed, it might occur secondary to iatrogenic injury to the superior gluteal nerve or gluteus medius muscle, adverse local tissue reactions, or osteolysis. Dr Alexa Pearce and colleagues present a review of the pros and cons of surgical reconstruction options for abductor insufficiency after total hip arthroplasty.

No gold standard exists for surgical repair of soft tissue in patients with knee replacement who have undergone multiple operations. Muscle flaps are often used by orthopedic and plastic reconstructive surgeons, but closed incisional negative pressure wound therapy might prove to be the best option in the long run. Dr Gerard A. Sheridan and colleagues report that a combination of those techniques, tailored to each patient, is likely to be the superior approach on multioperated knees.

Extensor mechanism disruptions are one of the most debilitating complications that can occur after total knee arthroplasty. Primary repair with and without augmentation as well as allograft reconstruction has been among the top surgical solutions, while synthetic grafts are showing promise for future patients. Drs Michael Bisogno and Giles Scuderi discuss an algorithm for treating these injuries, and they explore the surgical techniques for each approach.

In the trauma section, Dr Ahmed Mansour and colleagues review the fundamentals of reconstruction for lower-extremity wounds in limb salvage surgery and discuss the surgical techniques that can be applied broadly for lower-extremity wounds. Techniques for closing posttraumatic soft tissue wounds are the subject of an article by Dr James Blair and colleagues, who examine methods for skin closure, secondary wound closure, and rotational flaps of the lower leg. Split-thickness skin grafting, pie crusting, and negative pressure wound therapy are discussed,

as are rotational gastrocnemius, soleus, and reverse sural artery flaps. This review emphasizes techniques for nonvascular and nonmicrovascular orthopedic surgeons.

Cerebral palsy (CP) is the focus of the pediatric section in this issue. Patients with CP often present with hindfoot varus and dorsiflexion weakness, which can be corrected by tibialis posterior tendon transfer. Drs Lydia McKeithan and Amanda Whitaker describe the techniques and possible difficulties in successfully carrying out a tibialis posterior tendon transfer. They note that the foot and ankle must be flexible and lack skeletal deformity, and in order for the tendon transfer to function properly, electrical impulses of tibialis posterior should be present on electromyography during the swing phase of gait.

For the hand and wrist section, Dr Nicholas James and colleagues provide an overview of sagittal-band injuries, which can result in painful malalignment of the extensor tendon over the metacarpal heads as well as tendon subluxation or dislocation. If this kind of injury is discovered and treated within 3 weeks, surgery may not be necessary. If surgery is required, either direct repair or reconstruction of the sagittal band will restore anatomic alignment of the extensor tendon.

In arthroscopic shoulder stabilization surgery, remplissage, a nonanatomic capsulotenodesis of the infraspinatus tendon, is used to treat Hill-Sachs lesions in patients at increased risk of recurrent instability with isolated Bankart repair. This technique also has been suggested as a possible solution for patients after isolated anterior labral repair who are at high risk of recurrent instability. Several remplissage techniques have been developed, including a knotless method. Drs William Polio and Tyler Brolin review the history of the remplissage technique, the indications, and the improved patient outcomes compared with a standard Bankart repair.

Management of soft tissues is an important part of total shoulder arthroplasty (TSA). The success of any TSA also depends on proper release of the shoulder capsule and repair of the rotator cuff tendons. Drs Brandon Romero and John Horneff describe appropriate soft tissue techniques that will make the surgery easier and lead to better outcomes.

Orthop Clin N Am 53 (2022) xi–xii
https://doi.org/10.1016/j.ocl.2022.04.001
0030-5898/22/© 2022 Published by Elsevier Inc.

In the section on the foot and ankle, Dr James Jastifer provides a review of surgical repair of plantar-plate tears to stabilize the metatarsophalangeal (MTP) joint. During the last 10 years, much guidance has been published about how to treat MTP joint instability, which can cause metatarsalgia, usually in the second toe. Short-term outcomes of such surgeries have been good, but not great. Yet they show long-term promise in regard to pain relief and patient satisfaction.

As always, we thank these authors for contributing to the body of clinical knowledge that guides orthopedists in their treatment of patients around the world.

Frederick M. Azar, MD
Department of Orthopaedic Surgery and
Biomedical Engineering
University of Tennessee/Campbell Clinic
1211 Union Avenue, Suite 510
Memphis, TN 38104, USA

E-mail address:
fazar@campbellclinic.com

Knee and Hip Reconstruction

Diagnosis and Treatment Options of Abductor Insufficiency After Total Hip Replacement

Alexa N. Pearce, BA, Jeffrey B. Stambough, MD,
Simon C. Mears, MD, PhD, Charles Lowry Barnes, MD*,
Benjamin M. Stronach, MS, MD

KEYWORDS

- Abduction weakness • Instability • Total hip arthroplasty • Fatty infiltration • Chronic tears
- Trendelenburg • Muscle transfer • Tendon allograft

KEY POINTS

- Abductor insufficiency following total hip arthroplasty (THA) is a rare but serious condition that can result in recurrent hip instability.
- Patients typically present with a positive Trendelenburg sign, lateral hip pain, and abduction weakness that worsen in the lateral decubitus position; posterior dislocations may also occur.
- Reconstruction techniques are indicated for patients with chronic, irreparable tears; most notably, the gluteus maximus transfer has shown promising results for strength restoration and pain remediation.

INTRODUCTION

Abductor muscle insufficiency is a common cause of pain and disability after total hip arthroplasty (THA). This can be a spontaneous occurrence or traumatic avulsion of the greater trochanter (GT) or abductor insertion, as well as abductor tendinosis.[1–3] Severe abductor insufficiency is associated with advanced fatty muscle infiltration of the abductors.[4] Soft tissue deficiency is a major determinant in posterior instability following THA.[5] Diagnosis of abductor insufficiency can be difficult, and lateral hip pain is often thought to be trochanteric bursitis and ignored.[3] Primary repair is frequently not a viable option, as the diagnosis is often late, and chronic muscle atrophy and tissue retraction lead to poor results in repair.

This review discusses the cause and diagnosis of abductor insufficiency following THA. Workup including clinical examination and radiological findings are reviewed. The authors present surgical treatment options for reestablishing the integrity of the abductor complex with goals to improve pain, limp, and instability.

ANATOMY

The hip abductor muscle group originates on the ilium and includes the gluteus medius, gluteus minimus, and tensor fasciae latae (TFL). The posterior and anterior aspects of the gluteus medius insert on the lateral surface of the GT at the superior-posterior facet and lateral facet, respectively.[6] The gluteus minimus inserts on the anterior facet of the GT, and the TFL attaches to the iliotibial band. Together, these structures stabilize the hip during gait and facilitate hip internal rotation, external rotation, and abduction.[7] The gluteus maximus serves as an

---

Department of Orthopaedic Surgery, University of Arkansas for Medical Sciences, 4301 West Markham Street, Box 531, Little Rock, AR 72205, USA
* Corresponding author.
E-mail address: CLBarnes@uams.edu

Orthop Clin N Am 53 (2022) 255–265
https://doi.org/10.1016/j.ocl.2022.03.001
0030-5898/22/© 2022 Elsevier Inc. All rights reserved.

extensor rather than an abductor because of its attachments to the fascia lata and gluteal tuberosity rather than the GT.

The abductor muscles are innervated by the superior gluteal nerve (SGN), which extends through the sciatic foramen to the intermuscular plane of the gluteus medius and minimus muscles, terminating immediately after entering the TFL or continuing to the inferior aspect of the muscle.[8]

CAUSE OF ABDUCTOR MUSCLE DEFICIENCY

Intraoperative Trauma due to Surgical Approach

Surgical approach during THA is one of the most notable sources of direct damage to the abductor muscles or indirect muscle damage owing to innervation. The direct lateral (Hardinge) approach requires the splitting of the gluteus medius with mobilization of the anterior muscle and a segment of the anterior vastus lateralis.[9] Damage to the abductor muscle belly may result in heterotopic ossification or abductor weakness secondary to proximal migration of the abductor tendon or denervation of the anterior aspects of the abductor muscles.[10] Abductor repair during closure is another potential source of trouble, as these can be done with heavy nonabsorbable sutures or anchors into the anterior GT. If this does not heal or the patient experiences an early complication, this can lead to failure of repair and eventual abductor deficiency.

Failed Total Hip Arthroplasty

Degenerative processes affecting the muscle and/or bone following failed THA may also result in tendon avulsion and abductor insufficiency. Failure of THA, through bearing wear or infection, can prompt the osteolytic destruction of bone stock in the GT, resulting in chronic avulsion.[11,12] Fragmentation of the GT may cause the site of muscle attachment to move to an abnormal, fixed proximal position, an occurrence known as trochanteric escape.[11] If the proximal and distal attachment of the gluteus medius and vastus lateralis remains attached to the GT but the bony attachment to the femur is lost, the trochanteric fragment or fragments may migrate anteriorly owing to pull from the anterior gluteus medius fibers. Revision THA increases the risk for abductor insufficiency. With each additional surgery, the quality of soft tissue deteriorates, and further scar tissue develops, decreasing the possibility of reestablishing a stable joint owing to a disruption of soft tissue

tensioning. Lack of adequate soft tissue can result in the absence of the native capsule or postarthroplasty pseudocapsule, which normally serves as a stabilizing structure preventing dislocation.[13]

Metal-Associated Arthroplasty Failure

Abductor deficiency has also been linked to lymphocyte-dominated vasculitis-associated lesions and pseudotumors in patients with metal-on-metal, modular neck, or metal-on-polyethylene bearings.[14] Metal-associated THA may result in an adverse local tissue reaction (ALTR) that can lead to necrosis of bone, muscle, and soft tissue.[15]

Deficiency of the hip stabilizers may result both directly from ALTR and from revision THA following ALTR, which requires excision of necrotic tissue. Severe abductor insufficiency following revision of metal-on-metal THA has been cited as a risk factor for subsequent revision.[16]

Other Risk Factors

Further risk factors for abductor insufficiency following THA include cerebral dysfunction and prior spinal disease or surgery, the latter of which may result in the compression of the SGN.[17,18] Parkinson disease, postpolio syndrome, cerebral palsy, and stroke can also result in decreased strength and function of the hip stabilizers with resultant increased risk for dislocation.[19]

In addition, acute abductor insufficiency may occur following THA for tumor resection.[20] The lack of well-defined anatomic planes in this region allows for unconfined growth of tumors,[21] which may distort the soft tissues that stabilize the hip. Musculotendinous attachments and the SGN may thus be disturbed during tumor resection, particularly when en bloc removal of the abductor muscles is required.

PATIENT EVALUATION

Accurate diagnosis of abductor insufficiency is important for successful treatment. Clinical presentation typically includes a positive Trendelenburg sign, abductor lurch, lateral hip pain, and abductor weakness. A history of recurrent posterior dislocation is common. Imaging is important to eliminate other causes of instability and confirm the presence of abductor muscle tear and/or fatty infiltration with radiographs, MRI, and/or sonography.

Gait and Stance Analysis

Abductor deficiency has been correlated with a positive Trendelenburg sign, which is indicated by pelvic sag when the patient performs an ipsilateral one-legged stance (**Fig. 1**).[22] In a normal patient, contraction of the gluteus medius on the stance side allows for maintained elevation of the pelvis on the unsupported side.

The Trendelenburg sign is also considered positive if the patient is unable to maintain pelvic elevation for 30 seconds (fatigue test).[17] When the regular Trendelenburg test is negative and the fatigue test is positive, smaller tears may be present.[6]

Gait should also be assessed for abnormalities. Patients most often exhibit abductor lurch when walking,[22] with the trunk swaying to the contralateral side during the stance phase of the affected limb.[23] This is a compensatory mechanism whereby the patient is using their upper body weight to offset the pelvic obliquity caused by abductor insufficiency.

Finally, leg length discrepancy may lead to insufficient soft tissue tension or can cause a gait disturbance owing to gait imbalance and thus must be ruled out as a cause of abnormal gait when abductor deficiency is suspected. This can be achieved through assessment of overall leg lengths, pelvic obliquity, and spinal alignment.[17]

Lateral Hip Pain

One of the most significant symptoms of abductor insufficiency is lateral hip pain. GT pain syndrome encompasses trochanteric bursitis and other gluteal tendinopathies. The misdiagnosis of trochanteric bursitis is not uncommon in the setting of a gluteal tendon tear, but muscle damage is increasingly recognized as a source of pain over the GT in recent years.[24] Physicians should consider the possibility of abductor instability, opting for advanced

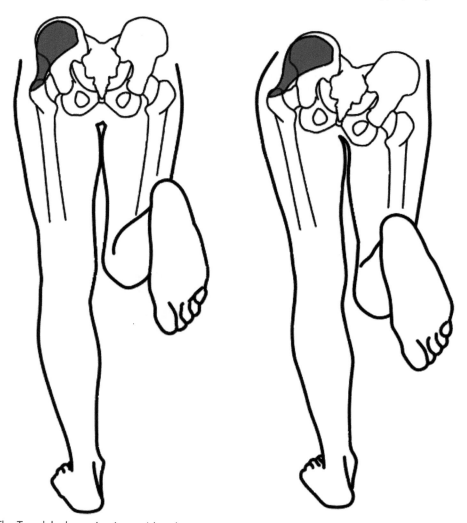

Fig. 1. The Trendelenburg sign is considered positive (*right*) when pelvic sag occurs.

imaging and examination maneuvers to rule out this pathologic condition.

Abductor Weakness and Decreased Range of Motion

An additional sign of abductor insufficiency is abduction weakness that worsens in a lateral decubitus position.[25] Passive muscle strength in the lateral position should be tested using the internal rotation lag sign, with the patient's knee flexed (45°) and their hip joint passively abducted. A positive sign occurs when internal rotation of the hip is painful or not possible, indicating potential lesions of the abductor muscle.[26]

Dislocation

Dislocation may occur as a result of posterior soft tissue deficiency. Dislocation occurs in up to 28% of THA revisions,[27] as compared with just 0.4% to 4.8% following primary THA.[18] This drastic increase in dislocation rate is often due to loss of soft tissue integrity with decreased musculature of the hip following revision surgery.[11]

Other factors that may lead to dislocation following THA include small femoral head diameter, elevated rim liners, deficient neck offset, low head-to-neck ratio, and component malposition.[28] Hyperlaxity syndrome, anterior-superior impingement, heterotopic bone impingement, posterior bursa presence, and socket dysplasia may result in dislocation as well.[5]

Additional risk factors for hip dislocation after THA include female sex, age greater than 70 years, trochanteric nonunion, neuromuscular disorders, and soft tissue imbalance.[13,28] Cognitive impairment may prevent adequate patient education, resulting in the execution of maneuvers that lead to dislocation. Ethanol use and medical comorbidities such as obesity also increase dislocation risk.[18,28]

Imaging
Radiographic findings

Radiographs are an essential component of the patient evaluation and include an anteroposterior pelvis and cross-table lateral hip radiograph at a minimum. Radiographs may help to eliminate other potential issues, including component loosening or malposition, trauma, impingement, or excessive wear that may account for symptoms.[3,19] Pathologic condition related to muscle deficiency can also be identified, such as osteolysis, trochanteric malunion or nonunion, and enthesophytes at the margin of the GT (Fig. 2).[19,24] Furthermore, tears of the abductor tendons or other tendinopathy

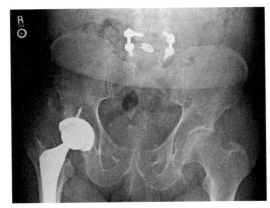

Fig. 2. Anteroposterior pelvic radiograph showing right THA with heterotopic ossification within the gluteus medius muscle and shortened right leg in comparison to the native hip.

can be suggested by surface irregularities of more than 2 mm at the insertion site.[29]

MRI findings

MRI has a reported accuracy of 91% in detecting gluteal tendon tears.[30] T1-weighted images with fat saturation, combined with axial T2-weighted images, are useful in identifying both partial and complete tears[24] (Fig. 3). When muscle atrophy has occurred, an increased signal at the site of tendon retraction can typically be seen.[31] MRI should be considered the gold standard for hip abductor muscle imaging. When metal implants are present, one should consider obtaining a metal artifact reductions sequence protocol.

In addition to identifying tears, MRI can reveal thickening, delamination, separation, retraction,

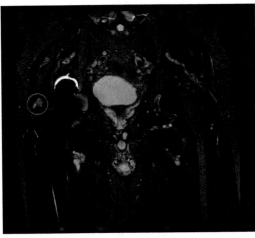

Fig. 3. T2 sequence MRI of the patient from Fig. 2 demonstrating gluteus medius tear of the right hip at the GT insertion with 3.5 cm of retraction (circle).

and fat saturation of the abductor tendons.[24] Atrophy and fatty degeneration can be graded using the Goutallier scale, with a score ≥ 2 constituting advanced fatty muscle degeneration (Table 1).[26] It should be noted that abductor insufficiency due to surgical approach typically demonstrates fatty infiltration without tendon detachment on MRI.[32]

Sonographic findings
The diagnosis of abductor muscle avulsion can be challenging with sonography owing to difficulty in identifying anatomic landmarks, but it provides useful information in regards to the soft tissues.[31] Partial-thickness tears are identifiable on sonogram as focal anechoic areas with no intact fibers or irregular hypoechoic bands within the substance of the tendon, whereas full-thickness tears can be seen as distinct bands spanning the full width of either abductor.[33]

Garcia and colleagues have noted certain advantages of sonography over MRI after THA, as sonography is not affected by metal artifact that can occur with MRI with the potential for poor resolution.[34] Other benefits of sonography are that it is cost-effective, widely available, radiation-free, and well-tolerated by patients.

Electromyography
Electromyography (EMG) can be used to confirm damage to the SGN[9] and thus may help rule out spinal pathologic condition as a cause of instability when surgery is being considered for abductor insufficiency. Coaxial-needle EMG reveals acute denervation as fibrillation potentials and/or positive acute waves within the SGN region of innervation.[9]

TREATMENT OPTIONS
Surgical Techniques
A variety of techniques have been described to treat abductor tendon deficiency. These include primary repair, allograft reconstruction, vastus lateralis transfers, trochanteric slide osteotomy (TSO), free flap, and gluteus maximus transfer. Prosthetic instability and implant loosening must also be addressed at the time of surgery. This may require component revision to improve the position of femoral or acetabular implants, increasing limb length and offset with longer heads, the use of large heads, dual mobility devices, and high offset or constrained liners.

Primary repair
Primary or direct repair of the abductors after THA is most successful when carried out at less than 15 months following the tear,[35] as patients with both partial- and full-thickness tears will have less muscular atrophy.[25] Primary repair of abductor tears is performed similarly to rotator cuff repair and can be carried out in an open or arthroscopic manner. Arthroscopic repair is typically only recommended for patients with low-grade tears,[36] as it does not allow the surgeon to evaluate the lateral surface of the tendon insertion site as readily as an open repair.[37]

In the open technique via lateral approach described by Lübbeke and colleagues,[35] the deep fascia is opened, and the abductor muscles are mobilized at the tendinous stumps. Approximately 5 nonabsorbable sutures are integrated into the tendon ends using a Bunnell-type technique and then passed through an equal quantity of transosseous tunnels.

There are several disadvantages to primary repair that must be considered. Fatty degeneration may persist following the procedure, predisposing patients to retear.[4] Indeed, direct repairs have a retear rate of 6% to 50% in the setting of late presentation after THA,[37] attributable in many cases to inadequate healing caused by poor tendon quality.[24] In addition, studies have shown primary repair to provide inconsistent results for pain relief and limp reduction.[38,39] In the setting of chronic tears with significant retraction or atrophy, or when surgical removal of the abductors is required in the setting of tumor, primary repair is typically not a viable treatment option,[38] and the surgeon should consider reconstruction methods, such as grafting techniques and/or muscle transfer.

Allograft reconstruction
An option for treating patients with abductor insufficiency is Achilles tendon allograft, which is indicated for patients who have undergone multiple revisions and have inadequate autogenous tissue for reconstruction using autologous

Table 1					
Classification of fatty infiltration according to the Goutallier scale					
Grade	0	1	2	3	4
Description	Normal muscle	Some fatty streaks	<50% fatty infiltration	Equal amounts fat and muscle	>50% fatty infiltration

tissue.[5,17] Numerous studies have shown that Achilles tendon allograft scan provides pain relief, improves gait and strength, and prevents dislocation.[3] The technique can be used when there is severe tendon loss, with or without muscular atrophy.[25] However, abductor muscle mass that shows contractility on electrical stimulation should be present.[3]

Fehm and colleagues[3] describe using a fresh-frozen Achilles tendon allograft with an osseous block beveled to dovetail into a trough made in the vastus ridge of the GT. The tendinous portion of the allograft is passed through the abductors and looped back on itself, then sutured to the gluteus minimus, the anterior capsule, and the posterior gluteus medius. The investigators found this technique was successful in substantially improving Harris hip and pain scores for 6 out of 7 patients at 24 to 48 months and increasing average abductor strength from 2.6 to 4.1 on the 5-point scale.[3]

van Warmerdam and colleagues[40] used an Achilles allograft sling technique in 3 different manners on patients with recurrent instability following THA: with a calcaneal bone wafer fixed to the ischium or to the GT, or with soft tissue graft alone sutured to soft tissue. Seven out of 8 patients experienced no further dislocations following the allograft. Disadvantages of tendon allografts include their cost and the dependence of their success on abductor muscle function.[1] This technique also places further nonautogenous material into the hip joint that can be problematic in regards to infection.

Vastus lateralis transfer

Vastus lateralis transfer is another salvage method for patients who have undergone multiple revisions and is particularly useful when there is a large separation between the gluteus medius tendon and the proximal femur.[17] A study by Kohl and colleagues[41] showed vastus lateralis transfer to be capable of providing pain relief, increasing strength, and improving ambulation.

Vastus lateralis transfer first requires the dissection and mobilization of the entire muscle from the rectus femoris with protection of the neurovascular pedicle proximally.[41] The distal insertion of the vastus lateralis is then separated from the confluence of the quadriceps. This entire mobilized section of vastus lateralis is then shifted proximally. The proximal vastus lateralis is then sutured into the remaining gluteus medius to reconstruct the abductors. The length of the vastus lateralis muscle is then stretched, and the distal portion of vastus lateralis is sutured back into the quadriceps insertion distally from which it was previously mobilized and released.

Advantages of the vastus lateralis shift include the limited restriction of hip flexion, the activation of the vastus lateralis in the same portion of the gait cycle as the abductor muscles, and the use of autogenous vascularized muscle for the reconstruction.[23] The separate neurovascular pedicle is an additional advantage, but there is a possibility of neurovascular damage secondary to overstretch of the neurovascular bundles.[23] Other disadvantages are the complexity of the procedure and the reduced strength of the quadriceps muscle.[23]

Trochanteric slide osteotomy

TSO is indicated in patients with an abductor complex that remains in continuity with the GT but with decreased muscular tension. One advantage of the TSO is that it can allow for preservation of the posterior capsule and short external rotators.[42] TSO is contraindicated for patients with osteolytic or osteopenic bone stock in the GT, as this can increase the risk for nonunion.[18]

TSO is typically carried out using a straight lateral incision to allow access to the anterior trochanter. An interval is created between the hip capsule and gluteus medius, and the posterior aspect of the vastus lateralis is incised 10 mm distal to the vastus ridge. The leg is placed in internal rotation, and the trochanter is osteotomized from just distal to the vastus ridge to just medial to the piriformis fossa in a similar manner used for surgical dislocation of the hip in the setting of trauma or femoroacetabular impingement. The gluteus medius inserts proximally into the trochanteric fragment, and the vastus lateralis inserts distally into the fragment. The fragment is slid distally to tension the abductors and can be shifted anteriorly or posteriorly as well depending on the specific problem being addressed. The fragment is then fixed with cables, wires, or sutures.[42]

Saadat and colleagues[18] achieved a success rate of 86% in using TSO to treat instability, confirming hopeful results from previous studies. However, a risk of nonunion following the procedure must be considered. A study by León and colleagues[43] found that osteotomies less than 10 cm were at risk for trochanter migration and suggested the use of a distal cerclage wire below the lesser trochanter to protect against such migration.

Free flap reconstruction: latissimus dorsi

Free neurovascular muscle transfer is another option for treating abductor insufficiency but is primarily used in acute cases when muscle deficiency is anticipated, such as in patients undergoing extensive tumor resection.[17] In the lower extremity, free muscle transfer has mainly been carried out following quadriceps tumor resection; however, several case reports have shown promising results for the use of this technique after hip abductor resection.[44,45] The main disadvantages of this treatment approach are the technical difficulty of the procedure and the potential for donor site morbidity.[38]

Gluteus maximus transfer

Gluteus maximus transfer for abductor reconstruction was originally described by Whiteside and colleagues[11] in 2006 and has since been used in both primary and revision THA, as well as in native hips.[22,46] This procedure should be considered for patients with chronic abductor tears, advanced fatty infiltration (>50%), or irreparable gluteus medius tears with more than 2 cm of retraction[4,17] (**Fig. 4**). For such circumstances, gluteus maximus transfer has been found to provide substantial pain relief and improvement in patient-reported outcomes.[4,12]

A functioning gluteus maximus is required for this treatment. The transfer uses the anterior portion of the gluteus maximus to reconstruct the gluteus medius and may incorporate a portion of the TFL and iliotibial band to aid in adduction and lend internal rotation strength.[22] A posterior flap from the gluteus maximus may also be used to reconstruct deficient external rotators and help provide stability.[26] As previously mentioned, the gluteus maximus is not an abductor itself because of its attachment to the fascia lata rather than the GT.[4] However, it is a convenient structure for reestablishing abduction strength because it is a large, powerful muscle that passes over the GT and has anterior

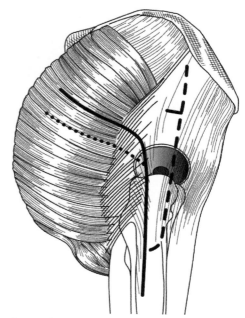

Fig. 5. A right hip depicting the initial deep incision made for the approach (*solid line*), the anterior flap (*heavy dashed line*), and the posterior flap (*dotted line*).

fibers that run nearly parallel to the femoral shaft when the muscle is in extension.[22] Furthermore, the muscle fibers of the gluteus maximus and TFL are closely aligned with one another.[22]

A posterolateral approach is used to access the gluteus maximus, which is subsequently split in its midsubstance in line with its fibers.[22] This requires an extensile approach proximally approaching the iliac crest and distally past the vastus ridge of the GT. The technique uses 2

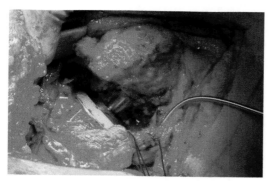

Fig. 4. : The GT with no evident remaining gluteus medius attachment after heterotopic ossification excision.

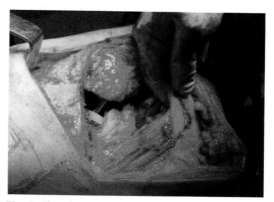

Fig. 6. The gluteus maximus is marked where the posterior flap will be developed. A small portion of fascia is included distally when possible to provide robust tissue for suturing into the transferred position.

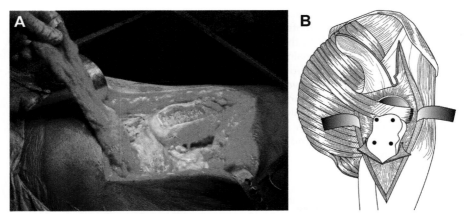

Fig. 7. (A) The posterior flap has been sutured into the anterior capsule and can be seen just superior to the GT. The trochanteric bone bed has been prepared to accept the anterior flap, and the anterior flap has been raised (being held in hand to the left of the image). The proximal portion of vastus lateralis has also been opened to accept the distal portion of the anterior flap. (B) The posterior flap is first sutured into the anterior capsule. The anterior flap (shown *curled back*) has been developed with drill holes placed in the GT with proximal vastus lateralis opening done to receive the anterior flap.

muscle flaps. The anterior flap uses anterior gluteus maximus along with a portion of the TFL and iliotibial band to reconstruct the gluteus medius and a posterior flap of gluteus maximus to reconstruct the external rotators (Fig. 5). The posterior flap is first developed (Fig. 6). This dissection extends toward the sciatic nerve, and it is important to locate and protect the nerve during this portion of the procedure.[22] The leg is gently abducted (15°) and maintained in this position for the remainder of the procedure. The posterior flap is then brought across the hip joint from posterior to anterior and sutured into anterior capsule under tension. This is performed before securing the anterior flap (used to re-create the gluteus medius) as the external rotator reconstruction will lie underneath the gluteus medius reconstruction. This flap will now be laying across the femoral neck superior to the GT.

The anterior triangular flap is then created using blunt and sharp dissection. A small horizontal notch is incised in the anterior portion of this flap proximally to allow for posterior excursion of the flap when it is attached to the GT. Next, the lateral surface of the GT (if present) is prepared using an osteotome for decortication to provide a cancellous bone bed for healing of the anterior flap, and holes are drilled in the cortical edges of the bone to secure the flap. A vertical 4- to 6-cm incision is made in line with the fibers of the vastus lateralis at the middle of the attachment site along the vastus ridge of the GT, and the proximal insertion of the vastus lateralis is detached from the femur

to create anterior and posterior triangular flaps of the proximal vastus lateralis (Fig. 7A, B). The muscle flap is sutured onto the GT (Fig. 8), and the distal tongue of the flap is secured in place under the vastus lateralis in a pants-over-vest fashion, closing the triangular flaps of the vastus lateralis down over the top of the distal portion of the muscle flap (Fig. 9A, B). This provides a supplementary soft tissue anchor point for this muscle flap in combination with the greater trochanteric attachment point. The posterior edge of the anterior flap is sutured to the top of the posterior flap for closure and further tensioning, and the remaining, intact portions of the fascia that were not harvested for the flaps are brought together and closed over the flaps distally. It is important to note that the anterior

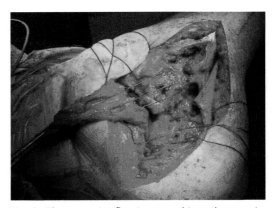

Fig. 8. The posterior flap is sutured into the anterior capsule; the anterior flap has been developed.

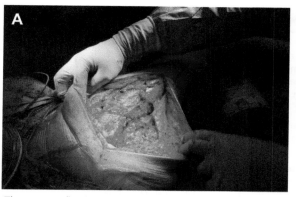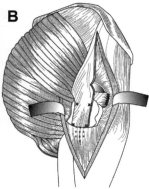

Fig. 9. (A) The anterior flap has been sutured onto the GT, and the vastus lateralis has been sutured over the distal portion of the flap in a pants-over-vest fashion to provide supplemental fixation. The intact iliotibial band and posterior portion of the gluteus maximus can be seen on the right side of the surgical exposure. (B) The anterior flap has been sutured onto the GT, and the triangular flaps of the vastus lateralis have secured over the distal end of the anterior flap in a pants-over-vest fashion.

limb of the anterior flap used to re-create the gluteus medius is left open to allow excursion (**Fig. 10**). In all, approximately one-half of the gluteus maximus is attached to the GT.

In the 2006 study by Whiteside and colleagues,[11] the above-described procedure was found to provide better pain relief in revision THA compared with leaving the trochanter unattached or excised. This pain relief may be attributable in part to the covering of a denuded GT with soft tissue, which also protects against local seroma and hematoma.[12,26] Quisquater and colleagues[12] found that the function of the abductor mechanism during stance and gait improved significantly in 44% of patients with severe defects following gluteus maximus transfer. In another

study, most muscle transfer patients demonstrated an improvement of 1 to 3 points on the 5-point muscle strength scale at last follow-up, as compared with preoperative values.[2]

Several disadvantages to the procedure exist. Most notably, its success is closely tied to the amount of preoperative abductor muscle degeneration. In addition, the possibility of osteopenic bone at the GT owing to stress shielding can make anchoring the muscle flap difficult.[12] In such cases, bone tunnels should be made deeper to provide an adequate bone bridge, and the distal vastus lateralis repair can be reinforced to help protect the trochanteric attachment.

Finally, at least one study has found that restoration of active abduction is poor and that the force vector for abduction is abnormal after the transfer.[26] However, Shea and colleagues[38] have noted that delayed return of active abduction may be due to the use of the gluteus maximus flap alone; thus, this phenomenon may be remedied by additional TFL transfer.

SUMMARY

Abductor deficiency is a serious concern following THA, leading to gait abnormality, severe pain, and hip instability. Careful clinical examination with adequate diagnostic imaging can help to pinpoint the cause of instability, especially in the case of abductor deficiency, which increases the chances of successful revision procedures. In the face of post-THA abductor-trochanteric compromise, abductor function may be adequately restored through several operative techniques, the most promising of which is the gluteus maximus transfer.

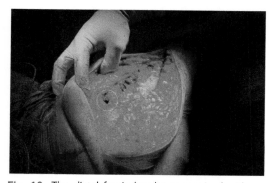

Fig. 10. The distal fascia has been repaired with suture, and the posterior fascia has been sutured to the posterior edge of the anterior flap. The horizontal incision previously made in the anterior edge of the fascia has allowed for posterior and distal excursion of the flap and is now seen as a hole in the anterior fascia (*circle*). This is intentionally left open to allow for muscular excursion with hip motion.

CLINICS CARE POINTS

- Abductor insufficiency secondary to abductor avulsion or fatty degeneration of the muscle following total hip arthroplasty is a rare but serious condition resulting in recurrent hip instability.

- Abductor avulsion occurs in less than 1% of patients following total hip arthroplasty.

- Abductor tears are suggested by a positive Trendelenburg sign; partial-thickness tears may be present if the Trendelenburg sign is negative, but the Trendelenburg fatigue test is positive.

- Abductor insufficiency is suggested by abductor weakness that worsens in the lateral decubitus position.

- Both abductor tears and fatty degeneration of the muscle can be identified with MRI and sonography.

- Surgical treatment is typically indicated for abductor insufficiency when nonsurgical means fail to adequately remediate pain and reestablish function.

- Primary repair is indicated for tears occurring within 15 months of primary total hip arthroplasty with little muscle atrophy and no trochanteric retraction.

- Reconstruction techniques are indicated for patients with chronic, irreparable tears; most notably, the gluteus maximus transfer has shown promising results for strength restoration and pain remediation.

REFERENCES

1. Chandrasekaran S, Darwish N, Vemula SP, et al. Outcomes of gluteus maximus and tensor fascia lata transfer for primary deficiency of the abductors of the hip. Hip Int 2017;27(6). https://doi.org/10.5301/hipint.5000504.

2. Kenanidis E, Kyriakopoulos G, Kaila R, et al. Lesions of the abductors in the hip. EFORT open Rev 2020;5(8). https://doi.org/10.1302/2058-5241.5.190094.

3. Fehm MN, Huddleston JI, Burke DW, et al. Repair of a deficient abductor mechanism with Achilles tendon allograft after total hip replacement. J Bone Joint Surg - Ser A 2010;92(13):2305–11.

4. Maldonado DR, Annin S, Chen JW, et al. Combined transfer of the gluteus maximus and tensor fasciae latae for irreparable gluteus medius tear using contemporary techniques. JBJS Open Access 2020;5(4):e20.00085. https://doi.org/10.2106/jbjs.oa.20.00085.

5. McGann WA, Welch RB. Treatment of the unstable total hip arthroplasty using modularity, soft tissue, and allograft reconstruction. J Arthroplasty 2001;16(8):19–23.

6. Davies JF, Stiehl JB, Davies JA, et al. Surgical treatment of hip abductor tendon tears. J Bone Joint Surg - Ser A 2013;95(15):1420–5.

7. Flack NAMS, Nicholson HD, Woodley SJ. The anatomy of the hip abductor muscles. Clin Anat 2014;27(2). https://doi.org/10.1002/ca.22248. New York, NY.

8. Flack NAMS, Nicholson HD, Woodley SJ. A review of the anatomy of the hip abductor muscles, gluteus medius, gluteus minimus, and tensor fascia lata. Clin Anat 2012;25(6). https://doi.org/10.1002/ca.22004. New York, NY.

9. Picado CHF, Garcia FL, Marques W. Damage to the superior gluteal nerve after direct lateral approach to the hip. Clin Orthopaedics Relat Res 2007;78(455):209–11.

10. Barber TC, Roger DJ, Goodman SB, et al. Early outcome of total hip arthroplasty using the direct lateral vs the posterior surgical approach. Orthopedics 1996;19(10).

11. Whiteside LA, Nayfeh T, Katerberg BJ. Gluteus maximus flap transfer for greater trochanter reconstruction in revision THA. Clin Orthopaedics Relat Res 2006;(453):203–10.

12. Quisquater L, Timmermans A, Vandenabeele F, et al. Gluteus maximus transfer as an augmentation technique for patients with severe abductor deficiency of the hip. Orthopedics 2020;43(4):E299–305.

13. Yang C, Goodman SB. Outcome and complications of constrained acetabular components. Orthopedics 2009;32(2):115.

14. Lash NJ, Whitehouse MR, Greidanus NV, et al. Delayed dislocation following metal-on-polyethylene arthroplasty of the hip due to "silent" trunnion corrosion. bone Jt J 2016;98-B(2). https://doi.org/10.1302/0301-620X.98B2.36593.

15. Klemt C, Smith EJ, Oganesyan R, et al. Outcome of dual mobility constructs for adverse local tissue reaction associated abductor deficiency in revision total hip arthroplasty. J arthroplasty 2020;35(12). https://doi.org/10.1016/j.arth.2020.06.043.

16. Bonner B, Arauz P, Klemt C, et al. Outcome of re-revision surgery for adverse local tissue reaction in metal-on-polyethylene and metal-on-metal total hip arthroplasty. The J arthroplasty 2020;35(6S). https://doi.org/10.1016/j.arth.2020.02.006.

17. Elbuluk AM, Coxe FR, Schimizzi Gv, et al. Abductor deficiency-induced recurrent instability after total hip arthroplasty. JBJS Rev 2020;8(1):e0164. https://doi.org/10.2106/JBJS.RVW.18.00164.

18. Saadat E, Diekmann G, Takemoto S, et al. Is an algorithmic approach to the treatment of recurrent dislocation after THA effective? Clin Orthopaedics Relat Res 2012;470(2):482–9. https://doi.org/10.1007/s11999-011-2101-x.

19. Su EP, Pellicci PM. The role of constrained liners in total hip arthroplasty. Clin orthopaedics Relat Res 2004;420. https://doi.org/10.1097/00003086-200403000-00017.

20. DeFrancesco CJ, Kamath AF. Abductor muscle necrosis due to iliopsoas bursal mass after total hip arthroplasty. J Clin orthopaedics Trauma 2015; 6(4). https://doi.org/10.1016/j.jcot.2015.05.002.

21. Soyfer V, Corn BW, Bickels J, et al. Primary high-grade soft-tissue sarcoma of the buttock: a rare but distinct clinical entity. Br J Radiol 2016; 89(1062). https://doi.org/10.1259/bjr.20151017.

22. Whiteside LA. Surgical technique: transfer of the anterior portion of the gluteus maximus muscle for abductor deficiency of the hip. Clin Orthopaedics Relat Res 2012;470(2):503–10.

23. Christofilopoulos P, Kenanidis E, Bartolone P, et al. Gluteus maximus tendon transfer for chronic abductor insufficiency: the Geneva technique. HIP Int 2020. https://doi.org/10.1177/1120700020924330.

24. Fox OJK, Wertheimer G, Walsh MJ. Primary open abductor reconstruction: a 5 to 10-year study. J Arthroplasty 2020;35(4):941–4.

25. Suppauksorn S, Nwachukwu BU, Beck EC, et al. Superior gluteal reconstruction for severe hip abductor deficiency. Arthrosc Tech 2019;8(10):e1255–61.

26. Ruckenstuhl P, Wassilew GI, Müller M, et al. Functional assessment and patient-related outcomes after gluteus maximus flap transfer in patients with severe hip abductor deficiency. J Clin Med 2020;9(6):1823.

27. Brooks PJ. Dislocation following total hip replacement: causes and cures. The bone Jt J 2013;95-B(11):67–9.

28. Ardiansyah Hadisoebroto I. Gluteus maximus transfer and mass graft (capsulorraphy) in recurrent hip dislocation with the history of total hip replacement: a case series. Int J Surg Case Rep 2021;82(71):105890.

29. Steinert L, Zanetti M, Hodler J, et al. Are radiographic trochanteric surface irregularities associated with abductor tendon abnormalities? Radiology 2010; 257(3). https://doi.org/10.1148/radiol.10092183.

30. Cvitanic O, Henzie G, Skezas N, et al. MRI diagnosis of tears of the hip abductor tendons (gluteus medius and gluteus minimus). AJR Am J roentgenology 2004; 182(1). https://doi.org/10.2214/ajr.182.1.1820137.

31. Twair A, Ryan M, O'Connell M, et al. MRI of failed total hip replacement caused by abductor muscle avulsion. AJR Am J roentgenology 2003;181(6). https://doi.org/10.2214/ajr.181.6.1811547.

32. Müller M, Tohtz S, Winkler T, et al. MRI findings of gluteus minimus muscle damage in primary total hip arthroplasty and the influence on clinical outcome. Arch orthopaedic Trauma Surg 2010; 130(7). https://doi.org/10.1007/s00402-010-1085-4.

33. Connell DA, Bass C, Sykes CJ, et al. Sonographic evaluation of gluteus medius and minimus tendinopathy. Eur Radiol 2003;13(6):1339–47.

34. Garcia Flavio Luis, et al. Sonographic evaluation of the abductor mechanism after total hip arthroplasty. Ultrasound Med 2010;29(3):465–71. https://doi.org/10.7863/jum.2010.29.3.465.

35. Lübbeke A, Kampfen S, Stern R, et al. Results of surgical repair of abductor avulsion after primary total hip arthroplasty. The J arthroplasty 2008; 23(5). https://doi.org/10.1016/j.arth.2007.08.018.

36. Voos JE, Shindle MK, Pruett A, et al. Endoscopic repair of gluteus medius tendon tears of the hip. Am J Sports Med 2009;37(4). https://doi.org/10.1177/0363546508328412.

37. Incavo SJ, Harper KD. Open hip abductor tendon repair into a bone trough: improved outcomes for hip abductor tendon avulsion. JBJS Essent Surg Tech 2020;10(2):1–14.

38. Shea GKH, Ching-HinYau R, Wai-Hung Shek T, et al. Transfer of the anterior gluteus maximus to address abductor deficiency following soft tissue tumour excision. J Orthopaedic Surg 2020;28(1):1–6.

39. Weber M, Berry DJ. Abductor avulsion after primary total hip arthroplasty. Results of repair. The J arthroplasty 1997;12(2). https://doi.org/10.1016/s0883-5403(97)90067-x.

40. van Warmerdam JM, McGann WA, Donnelly JR, et al. Achilles allograft reconstruction for recurrent dislocation in total hip arthroplasty. The J arthroplasty 2011;26(6). https://doi.org/10.1016/j.arth.2010.12.014.

41. Kohl S, Evangelopoulos DS, Siebenrock KA, et al. Hip abductor defect repair by means of a vastus lateralis muscle shift. The J arthroplasty 2012;27(4). https://doi.org/10.1016/j.arth.2011.06.034.

42. Sundaram K, Siddiqi A, Kamath AF, et al. Trochanteric osteotomy in revision total hip arthroplasty. EFORT open Rev 2020;5(8). https://doi.org/10.1302/2058-5241.5.190063.

43. León SA, Mei XY, Sanders EB, et al. Does trochanteric osteotomy length affect the amount of proximal trochanteric migration during revision total hip arthroplasty? The J arthroplasty 2019;34(11). https://doi.org/10.1016/j.arth.2019.06.034.

44. Ihara K, Kishimoto T, Kawai S, et al. Reconstruction of hip abduction using free muscle transplantation: a case report and description of the technique. Ann Plast Surg 2000;45(2). https://doi.org/10.1097/00000637-200045020-00015.

45. Barrera-Ochoa S, Collado-Delfa JM, Sallent A, et al. Free neurovascular latissimus dorsi muscle transplantation for reconstruction of hip abductors. Plast Reconstr Surg - Glob Open 2017;5(9). https://doi.org/10.1097/GOX.0000000000001498.

46. Thaunat M, Roberts T, Bah A, et al. Endoscopic transfer of gluteus maximus and tensor fascia lata for primary hip abductor deficiency. Arthrosc Tech 2020;9(9). https://doi.org/10.1016/j.eats.2020.04.024.

Soft Tissue Procedures in the Multiply Operated on Knee Replacement Patient

Gerard A. Sheridan, MD, FRCS[a,*],
Peter A. Lennox, MD, FRCS[b], Bassam A. Masri, MD, FRCS[a]

KEYWORDS

• Revision TKA • Incision • Soft tissue • Muscle flap • ciNPWT • Sham incision

---

KEY POINTS

• The medial gastrocnemius flap (MGF) success rate is 81% in the setting of deep soft tissue defect after complex primary or revision total knee arthroplasty (TKA). The success-limiting factor is the recurrence of infection more so than any inherent issue with flap functioning.
• Multiple surgeries of 5 or more have been shown to be associated with a significantly higher rate of implant failure and amputation in the setting of MGF.
• Closed incision negative pressure wound therapy seems to be more useful in the setting of revision hip and knee arthroplasty but harmful in the primary TKA setting.

INTRODUCTION

The options for soft tissue management around the knee in the revision knee replacement setting have been well documented and range from simple techniques such as delayed primary closure, healing by secondary intention and vacuum-assisted closure to more complex techniques requiring the input of a specialist plastic surgeon such as skin grafting, local flap coverage, and distant microsurgical tissue transfer.[1]

In the multiply operated on knee, the host soft tissue envelope is often more challenging to manage surgically when compared with a primary total knee arthroplasty (TKA) procedure. In the setting of infection, it has been shown that the need for soft tissue coverage when undergoing a gold standard 2-stage revision procedure is associated with a higher rate of recurrent infection after prosthesis reimplantation.[2] Pelt and colleagues also highlighted the risks associated with surgery after multiple previous interventions on knee replacements. It was shown

that knees that underwent 4 or more additional operations after the primary TKA were at significantly higher risk of failure.[2]

In this review, we explore in detail the role of soft tissue flaps, soft tissue expanders, sham incisions, and closed incision negative pressure wound therapy (ciNPWT). Each technique has its own specific benefits and significant considerations, which may be applied to the often uniquely challenging cases seen in the multiply operated on knee replacement.

Clinical Challenges

A spectrum of soft tissue challenges exists in the revision TKA setting. First, determining the location of the revision incision when multiple incisions are already present is paramount. The vascular supply to the anterior knee tissues predominantly originates from the medial aspect of the knee. For this reason, the most recent or the most lateral incision is used in order to prevent the catastrophic complication of full thickness wound necrosis (**Fig. 1**).[3] In addition to this approach, wide skin bridges of at least 8 cm

---

[a] Department of Orthopaedics, University of British Columbia, Vancouver, British Columbia, Canada;
[b] Department of Surgery, Division of Plastic and Reconstructive Surgery, University of British Columbia, Vancouver, British Columbia, Canada
* Corresponding author.
E-mail address: sheridga@tcd.ie

Orthop Clin N Am 53 (2022) 267–276
https://doi.org/10.1016/j.ocl.2022.03.004

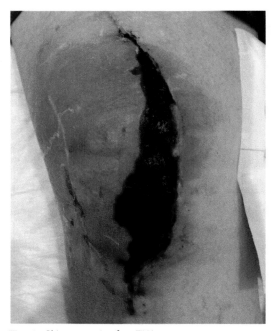

Fig. 1. Skin necrosis after TKA.

between incisions are recommended in the revision setting. Skin necrosis may lead to deep and catastrophic prosthetic joint infection. If there is no doubt about skin viability, a sham incision may be made without exposing the tissue deep to the capsule. The risks and benefits of sham incisions will be discussed later in this article.

Sinus tract formation often involves the prosthetic joint deep to the capsule and, by definition, constitutes a deep prosthetic joint infection. In this setting, not only is it necessary to undergo revision surgery for infection eradication but subsequent skin closure of the knee

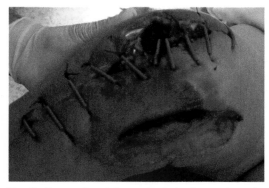

Fig. 2. Exposed metal prosthesis in the setting of a major soft tissue defect requiring revision TKA with the aid of a soft tissue flap for coverage.

may also be challenging. Complete sinus excision is essential in this case potentially creating the problem of inadequate skin availability for a tension-free closure. If a 2-stage surgical reimplantation approach with articulating spacer is adopted, the success rates for infection eradication in the setting of a preexisting sinus tract can be promising as demonstrated by Qui and colleagues.[4] In that article, 10 patients underwent a 2-stage reimplantation with articulating spacer and 9 of the 10 successfully achieved complete infection eradication at a mean of 50 months follow-up. Wound closure for these cases, especially in the revision hip and knee arthroplasty setting, may be significantly enhanced by the use of ciNPWT. Vacuum dressing techniques are simple and effective, especially in the setting of revision hip and knee arthroplasty.

After traumatic injuries, such as tibial plateau fractures and other periarticular fractures, skin adherence and soft tissue atrophy at the time of revision surgery may be problematic for adequate incision closure and protection of the implant while the wound is healing.[3] This issue may be managed using soft tissue expanders around the knee, with or without a local flap, before the knee replacement. The preoperative expansion techniques provide excess skin that may be recruited at the time of closure in the revision TKA setting. These expanders come with their own risks of infection, displacement and rupture as will be illustrated.

On the most severe end of the spectrum, there may be complete tissue loss over the prosthesis leading to exposure of the component (Fig. 2). In these circumstances, soft tissue coverage is the main clinical challenge. This may only be achieved with the use of either local or distant soft tissue flaps using the expertise of a plastic surgeon. The medial gastrocnemius flap (MGF) is the most common flap used in this setting but there are many alternatives that may be used depending on local anatomy and the specific characteristics of the soft tissue envelope in question.

The importance of mastering these salvage techniques to avoid either a recurrence of infection or failure of soft tissue closure, in which case amputation or chronic suppression with antibiotics become the only viable options for clinical management.

Surgical Techniques Available
Closed incision negative pressure wound therapy
Background. Negative Pressure Wound therapy is a well-described technique that has been applied to a wide number of specialties to

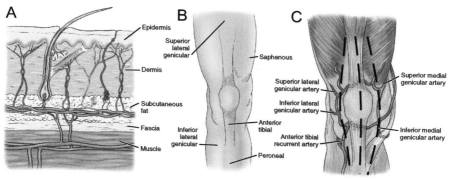

Fig. 3. Vascular supply to the skin around the knee. (*A*) Vascular supply to layers of the skin. (*B*) Arterial territories around the knee. (*C*) Incision location in relation to vascular supply.

improve wound healing through negative pressure.[5–7] NPWT creates a pressure gradient from within a wound to the outer environment, thereby reducing the likelihood of several risks. Such risks include the introduction of microorganisms into the wound and the formation of large static hematomas that may become a nidus for infection. NPWT also encourages microvascular formation in the area, which in turn improves the healing potential of the wound.

Recent level 1 evidence by Ailaney and colleagues, describing the results of a meta-analysis of randomized controlled trials, demonstrated that ciNPWT significantly reduced the risk of surgical site infections when compared with conventional dressings specifically in revision THA and TKA.[8] ciNPWT was also shown to significantly reduce the length of hospital stay and the need for reoperation in that study. However, noninfectious complications (specifically wound blistering) were significantly increased in primary TKA; therefore, the utility of this technique in the primary TKA setting is questionable at best.

The role for ciNPWT in revision hip and knee arthroplasty has also been demonstrated by Newman and colleagues.[9] In this study, 160 patients undergoing elective revision arthroplasty were prospectively randomized to receive either ciNPWT or a silver-impregnated occlusive dressing after surgery in a single institution. It was found that the postoperative wound complication rate in the control cohort was 23.8% versus 10.1% in the ciNPWT cohort (*P* = .022).

Other advantages associated with the use of ciNPWT include the financial gain to be made by institutions using this technique. In the setting of revision TKA, Pagani and colleagues demonstrated that ciNPWT is cost-effective at both high and low initial infection rates, across a broad range of treatment costs, and at inflated product expenses.[10] A recent systematic review and meta-analysis noted that in high-risk revision TKA and selected primary TKA cases, ciNPWT reduced wound complications and may have health-care cost savings also.[11]

2: SHAM INCISIONS
Knee Vascularity
An eloquent description of the considerations around surgical exposures in revision TKA is given by Younger and colleagues in their 1998 article.[12] The vascular supply to the skin around the knee is provided from a deep anastomosis just superficial to the deep fascia (**Fig. 3**). This anastomosis is mostly formed of vessels originating from the medial side of the knee joint from the saphenous artery and the descending genicular artery. For this reason, tissue flaps should be elevated deep to the distal extension of scarpa fascia, and not superficially, because there is little communication between vascular territories in the deep layers. This is relevant for the multiply operated knee, which may have numerous incisions in various and often conflicting locations. Poor placement of the incision used to gain access during revision knee surgery can predispose to superficial or full thickness skin necrosis and wound breakdown with catastrophic soft tissue complications and potential amputation.

To avoid these complications from developing, consultation with a plastic surgeon before surgery is imperative. In general, crossing previous transverse incisions at a 90° angle will not lead to any significant tissue compromise. Any angle created less than 60°, however, does introduce the risk of a tissue viability complication. In the presence of oblique incisions, the surgical incision can be curved to intersect the incision at 90°, instead of relying on the obliquity of the existing incision. For example, **Fig. 4** shows

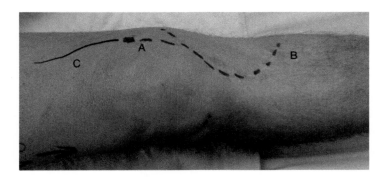

Fig. 4. Multiple knee incisions.

2 existing incisions marked by 2 dashed lines, A and B. It would have been best if the previous surgeon had planned incision A to intersect incision B at a right angle. For a knee replacement, incision A needs to be incorporated into the surgical incision C, with the understanding that its intersection with the previous incision B is not ideal.

Surgical Technique

One approach to deal with this challenging issue includes the use of sham incisions. Sham incisions are made through the planned skin-incision trajectory down as deep as the fascial layer but not through the fascial layer. They work based on the well-described plastic surgical principles of flap delay. The benefits of this incision are 2-fold: First, if the skin incision breaks down, a deep infection has been avoided because the deep fascia has not been breached. Second, creating flaps will promote collateral vascular formation in the region, which further increases the likelihood of incision healing at the time of the definitive revision TKA.[12]

Clinical Outcomes

Although sham incisions have been recognized by the arthroplasty community as a viable option in approaching complex revision cases with concerns for soft tissue healing, there is very little data to report on the effectiveness, outcomes, and complication profile of using this technique.[13,14] The complications associated with sham incisions include general perioperative risks such as anesthetic cardiorespiratory perioperative complications, postoperative venous thromboembolic disease, and local surgical site infection. The most concerning surgical outcome would be skin necrosis and soft tissue compromise. Even though a potential deep prosthetic joint infection has been avoided in this case, this complication still incurs significant morbidity

to the patient that may require further surgical intervention. Current evidence is unable to advise on the rate of skin necrosis in the setting of a sham incision before revision TKA. This is an area of the literature, which needs more attention in future research efforts.

Future Directions

Sham incisions are likely to remain in the armamentarium of the orthopedic surgeon required to perform complex revision TKA. However, well-designed studies are required to ensure that this technique is truly beneficial for patients with an acceptable complication profile. One potential use is at the time of hardware removal when the hardware cannot be safely removed at the time of knee replacement.

3: SOFT TISSUE EXPANDERS

Indications and Surgical Techniques

Soft tissue expansion involves the introduction of a subcutaneous device superficial to the patella and patellar tendon. The aim of this technique is to sequentially expand the skin overlying the anterior aspect of the knee joint in an effort to improve the mobility of soft tissue flaps created during the approach to the multiply operated on knee joint. The excess skin created over the time of expansion can be used to accommodate an increase in knee joint range of motion.

The early use of soft tissue expanders was applied to this clinical scenario specifically. A case series of 2 arthrodesis cases was reported in 1994 by Mahomed and colleagues.[15] The first case in this series underwent knee fusion after multiple knee operations and eventual development of septic arthritis. The other case underwent arthrodesis for severe osteoarthritis. In both cases, achievement of full postoperative flexion was a significant concern leading the treating surgeon to insert a soft tissue expander before the conversion procedure. Mahomed and colleagues report that in both cases, a postoperative flexion of 90° was reached, supporting the use of soft tissue expanders for conversion of arthrodesis cases.

Clinical Outcomes and Complications

A more recent case series of 2 cases demonstrates the widening indications for soft tissue expander usage and the alternative techniques that may be used.[16] Piuzzi and colleagues described their results of 2 cases where 2 separate single remote port tissue expanders were inserted subcutaneously into a single knee along the medial and lateral aspects of the proximal third of the lower leg. Both expanders were 700 mL in capacity. Two weeks after insertion, inflation with normal saline commenced at a rate of 10% of the expander volume. Monitoring consisted of capillary refill assessment of the overlying skin and observation of whether the patient could tolerate the procedure or not.

The first case was a 43-year-old man with severe posttraumatic arthritis after tibial plateau fracture requiring fixation leading to infection, external fixation, and ultimately hardware removal due to persistent infection. In this case, the lateral expander became infected requiring removal, debridement, and antibiotic treatment. The medial expander was preserved and after control of the lateral infection, medial expansion began. Thirteen months after the insertion of the tissue expanders, a TKA was performed with a MGF for coverage. The wound was closed using direct primary closure of the subcutaneous layers with skin staples for superficial closure. This particular case developed some significant complications including a neuroma of the internal saphenous nerve requiring excision and a deep prosthetic joint infection requiring a full 2-stage revision. The infection was ultimately cleared with satisfactory results achieved. Clearly, these are case reports, and firm conclusions cannot be drawn from isolated case reports. However, this illustrates that all options need to remain open, and the expertise of a plastic surgeon needs to be sought at the planning stages of these procedures, as opposed to when a problem arises.

The largest series of soft tissue expanders for TKA reported in the literature consists of 64 expansions for 59 cases.[17] Long and colleagues reported their experience during a 15-year period. The commonest indication for soft tissue expansion was the presence of conflicting incisions (n = 59) made from prior procedures followed by angular deformity (n = 5). The average number of previous operations per patient was 3.5, the average number of expanders used was 2.1, the average total volume per patient was 359 mL, and the process took an average of 70 days (range 36–174). In this series, minor complications were those that required local care only and major complications were those that required a return to the operating room. For this series, there were minor complications in 22% and major complications in 11% of cases. The minor complications consisted of 4 blisters, 6 cases of skin erythema, 1 wound breakdown, 1 shift in the position of the expander, 1 lateral skin breakdown, and 1 medial expander leakage. The major complications in this series included presumed expander displacement, infection over 1 of 4 expanders, 2 cases of swelling over the expanders, infection and skin breakdown, migration of tissue expanders, and 1 case of eschar formation over the expander with full thickness soft tissue loss.

Reporting on a series of 29 knees, Manifold and colleagues describe a minor complication rate of 21% after soft tissue expansion and 18% after the TKA procedure. These minor complications included skin blistering in 3 cases and erythema of the overlying skin in 3 cases also. The single major complication occurred in a patient who underwent radiation therapy to the area. Significant skin necrosis occurred requiring skin grafting. The patient did not proceed to TKA after this. Five patients experienced minor complications after TKA had been performed. These included 3 cases of postoperative incision drainage and 2 cases of hematoma formation.

Future Directions

In general terms, soft tissue expansion in the lower extremity has a very-high complication rate and is rarely done. Most plastic surgeons would avoid this around a TKR and would proceed directly to flap coverage. The superior outcomes of flaps and other plastic surgery techniques have made the use of expanders almost obsolete and mostly of historical significance.

4: SOFT TISSUE FLAPS

Introduction

Local, regional, and distant soft tissue flaps have provided many options to the plastic and orthopedic surgeons managing severe soft tissue defects in the context of the multiply operated TKA. The decision regarding which flap to use often depends on several factors including wound size and location, prosthetic infection status, patient comorbidity, and surgeon skillset.

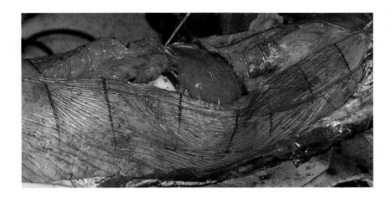

Fig. 5. MGF coverage for TKA components.

Many reconstructive options exist including perforator flaps, fasciocutaneous muscular flaps, and free microvascular flaps.[18]

The workhorse flap has been the local rotational MGF (Fig. 5). This flap is a particularly attractive option for the reconstructive plastic and orthopedic surgeon because this muscle provides a large mass that may be easily rotated to cover defects over the anteromedial aspect of the knee joint. This flap may not be appropriate for more lateral defects over the knee; however, a lateral gastrocnemius flap is possible, although the size of the lateral gastrocnemius muscle is smaller, and hence its reach may not be as long. It is ideal for covering large sinus tracks laterally that cannot be closed primarily.

Results of the Medial Gastrocnemius Flap

A recent systematic review, examining 16 studies, reports the success rate of the MGF to be 81% (195/241 patients) in the setting of a deep soft tissue defect after complex primary or revision TKA.[19] In this systematic review by Coombs and colleagues, the MGF success rate was not as high as the success rate for the fasciocutaneous flap coverage that was performed in 84 patients. The success rate of the fasciocutaneous flap coverage was reported at 90%. Patients undergoing delayed and prophylactic reconstruction in this study were reported to have equivalent success rates to the MGF at 81%.

The use of MGFs in the management of prosthetic TKA infection can be challenging. A retrospective review of 43 prosthetic TKA infections with associated soft tissue defects and managed with MGFs reported an infection-free survival rate of 71% at 2 years and 63% at 5 years.[20] Of these 43 cases, 4 did not undergo reimplantation, 11 received an arthrodesis implant, and the rate of subsequent amputation was 16%

with a mortality rate of 26% at follow-up. In this study, the only risk factor for reinfection was the Charlson Comorbidity Index. It should be noted that there were no failures of the flaps themselves. Tetreault and colleagues also reported on the use of MGFs in the context of prosthetic TKA infections and soft tissue defects. Thirty-one MGFs were used for soft tissue coverage over an infected TKA at a single institution during 8 years. Although there were no flap-related complications, the rate of reinfection was high at 52%. Implant survivorship at 4 years was 48% and 12 patients had a total of 19 reoperations in the period.[21] An even higher rate of reinfection rate of 69.2% at a mean follow-up of 3.3 years is reported by Warren and colleagues in their review of 26 consecutive patients undergoing rotational muscle flap surgery for full-thickness anterior soft tissue defect during the treatment of an infected TKA.[22] In all studies, the success-limiting factor is the recurrence of infection more so than any inherent issue with flap functioning. This is promising regarding the utility of this technique but the implications of undergoing this complex surgery only to fail due to reinfection are significant and should be well considered before performing this procedure.

The largest study to date reports on 83 patients where an MGF was used to cover the site of a primary or revision TKA. Houdek and colleagues report 10-year survival rates of 32% and 10-year amputation rates of 21%.[23] The risk of implant failure in this setting was significantly increased by severe obesity (BMI >40) and 5 or more prior surgical interventions on the knee. Amputation risk was also significantly increased when 5 or more prior procedures had been performed on the knee. A wound size of 50 cm or more and patients aged 65 years and older had a significantly higher risk of amputation also.[23] Although the overall rates of survival and amputation may reflect the complexity of comorbidity and infection in the multiply operated knee, flap coverage and function do not seem to be the problematic issues for this particular cohort, which bodes well for the continued application of this reconstructive technique.

Other Techniques

- Vastus Medialis and Lateralis

When an MGF is not possible (eg, in the case of very lateral defects, inadequate gastrocnemius muscle mass, or very large soft tissue defects), other regional coverage options may be explored. Many of these techniques are in their infancy and others are experimental. The distally based vastus lateralis is an example of a flap that provides local coverage without the need for microsurgical anastomosis. A small cohort of 4 cases (3 in a multiple-revised TKA and 1 post-traumatic amputation) reported skin closure in all 4 cases.[24] This is a technique rarely used but may provide an alternative option in the case where an MGF is not an option. This particular technique had issues with distal marginal necrosis and poor postoperative range of motion at a mean of 45°.

Vastus lateralis and vastus medialis have also been used as an adjunct to gastrocnemius and soleus to cover significant anterior soft tissue defects in the knee where the extensor mechanism is deficient. Whiteside and colleagues described their experience with this technique in their report of 8 patients. Four had vastus medialis transfer, 2 had vastus medialis and lateralis transfer, whereas 2 had medial vastus transfer. These transfers were combined with the regular gastrocnemius or soleus transfers.[25] All cases proceeded to heal the arthrotomy without any synovial leakage. Mean extensor lag was 22° and no flaps developed necrosis. Although these techniques are reported in low numbers, their initial results at least support their utility in the context of the multiple operated on TKA.

- Latissimus Dorsi

When locoregional options are not available, such as defects over the patella, free flaps may be considered. One such option is the latissimus dorsi (LD) free flap. This muscle is regularly used as a free flap for soft tissue coverage in a wide variety of anatomic locations.[26] Hierner and colleagues describe their results with its usage in 14 patients (4 of whom had a completely deficient extensor mechanism).[27] LD transfer occurred

simultaneously with the knee arthroplasty procedure in these patients. Skin breakdown occurred in 5 out of 14 patients. Four of these patients underwent grafting and 1 underwent a revision flap. Primary wound healing was achieved in 8 patients. Infection recurrence with ultimate conversion to arthrodesis occurred in 3 patients.

Recent evidence from a cohort of 18 patients undergoing revision TKA with an LD flap in the context of a multiple-revised TKA shows a 5-year implant survival of 75%.[28] Of the 18 patients treated for infection at a median follow-up of 49 months, 7 were infection-free, 7 were on suppressive antibiotics and 4 underwent above knee amputations. Again, the utility of free muscle flaps in the setting of a multiple-revised TKA is shown. Soft tissue coverage is possible but good function and infection eradication can be difficult to achieve in this challenging clinical setting.

- Prophylactic Flaps

In an effort to preempt any soft tissue compromise after TKA surgery, some authors have explored the role of prophylactic flap reconstruction of the knee before TKA. The advantages of this approach include the ability to achieve complete healing of an adequate soft tissue envelope before TKA instead of risking an issue with soft tissue healing with the simultaneous insertion of sterile metal TKA components. Casey and colleagues report their experience with the use of prophylactic flap reconstruction of the knee before TKA.[29] In this study, 23 patients were treated with TKA after a prophylactic flap reconstruction and 18 were treated with soft tissue flap reconstruction for a complication after TKA. For the prophylactic group, there was a 48% complication rate but all flaps survived after the TKA procedure took place. For the salvage flap reconstructions, 3 of the 18 patients ultimately required amputation to manage their complications. The negative aspect of a prophylactic approach is the requirement for multiple-staged procedures, which prolong the recovery time for each patient undergoing this management approach. After a prophylactic flap, the orthopedic surgeon has to take great care in raising the flap in order to not disrupt its blood supply. These flaps are often covered with a skin graft. The surgeon should identify where the blood supply to the flap is, and should make an incision and raise the flap in a manner that does not disturb its blood supply. For example, a MGF should be raised from lateral to medial, and the incision along a lateral gastrocnemius flap should be made along its medial side. In the case of a free flap over the anterior aspect of the knee, the incision should be made along its lateral side to avoid injuring the anastomosis medially from the femoral artery. Alternatively, involving the operating plastic surgeon in flap elevation for future procedures is an option.

The use of perforator flaps (eg, a local island medial sural artery perforator flap) in the prophylactic setting has been described in 2021 by Azoury and colleagues.[30] Seven patients undergoing single perforator flaps were included for the analysis. Three patients underwent local island medial sural artery perforator flaps, whereas the remaining 4 underwent anterolateral thigh (ALT) perforator free flaps. All flaps survived in all cases. One ALT flap patient developed a prosthetic joint infection requiring revision surgery but implant salvage was possible and the flap survived in all 7 cases. Perforator flaps have the added benefit that the majority are fasciocutaneous and therefore do not sacrifice any muscle function. Perforator flaps are becoming much more common and will likely be an increasingly used tool for soft tissue coverage.

SUMMARY

Soft tissue management in the multiply operated on knee can pose a multitude of challenges for both orthopedic surgeons and plastic surgeons alike. Although there are many surgical techniques that may be used in an effort to achieve a sterile, functional revision knee replacement, each technique has its specific disadvantages and no approach is without the potential for significant complication.

Preoperative assessment continues to be the most important first step. Assessing where any existing incisions are, and planning new incisions to incorporate these or minimize devascularization, is key to avoiding these devastating complications in the first place. Preoperative consultation with a plastic surgeon in complicated revision cases should also be considered.

One of the commonest approaches has been the MGF. Although still very useful, the largest reports on long-term survival report 10-year survival rates of 32% and 10-year amputation rates of 21%, not because of the presence of the flap but because of the underlying conditions leading to the need for the flap in the first place. Multiple operations of 5 or more have been shown to be associated with a significantly higher rate of implant failure and amputation. A poor prognosis should be communicated when patients meet the threshold of 5 or more multiple surgeries, although failure is by no means guaranteed. Many other flaps exist when the workhorse MGF is not appropriate for use.

The use of prophylactic flaps shows a similar amputation rate in the small studies reporting on these outcomes. Future large-scale studies may differentiate between the effectiveness of prophylactic and simultaneous flap coverage but currently no difference in clinical outcomes can be demonstrated.

Soft tissue expanders are less frequently used with less evidence available to support them. Sham incisions (delay procedure) provide a theoretically attractive option in that they avoid the risk of potential skin necrosis and deep infection after component reimplantation by virtue of adopting a staged approach. However, there is a significant paucity of evidence to advise on the actual rates of skin necrosis and so the exact role that sham incisions should play in the future of complex revision TKA is still unclear.

ciNPWT has shown to be effective in the revision THA and TKA setting, associated with significantly lower rates of wound complications when compared with other wound closure methods. This is a financially attractive option but it should be reserved for revision hip and knee arthroplasty only because it may be associated with significant skin complications, particularly in the primary TKA setting.

At the present time, no one technique is vastly superior to another. The most extensive literature available is in relation to muscle flaps, which will likely continue to be the workhorse technique for orthopedic and plastic reconstructive surgeons for the foreseeable future. ciNPWT may prove to be a superior method in time but further large-scale studies are required to expand our understanding of this technique. The continued use of a combination of these techniques, tailored to the specific patient, is likely to be the best approach to the complex problem of the multiply operated on knee into the future.

CLINICS CARE POINTS

- The medial gastrocnemius flap (MGF) is the most common flap used in the knee with multiple interventions.

- The MGF success rate is 81% in the setting of deep soft tissue defect after complex primary or revision TKA. The success-limiting factor is the recurrence of infection more so than any inherent issue with flap functioning.
- Multiple surgeries of 5 or more have been shown to be associated with a significantly higher rate of implant failure and amputation in the setting of MGF.
- The success rate of the fasciocutaneous flap coverage has been reported as high as 90%.
- Prophylactic and simultaneously performed flaps have similar success rates in the revision TKA setting.
- Complication rates with soft tissue expanders range from 33% to 39%.
- Sham incisions have an insufficient body of evidence to either support or refute their usage in the surgical management of soft tissues in the multiply operated on knee.
- Closed incision negative pressure wound therapy (ciNPWT) seems to be more useful in the setting of revision hip and knee arthroplasty but harmful in the primary TKA setting.
- ciNPWT is financially viable and will likely continue to provide a useful option for both orthopedic and plastic surgeons involved with managing the multiply operated on knee.
- Preoperative assessment and consideration of plastic surgical consultation should be considered in complex revision patients.

DISCLOSURE

The authors have nothing to disclose.

REFERENCES

1. Rao AJ, Kempton SJ, Erickson BJ, et al. Soft tissue reconstruction and flap coverage for revision total knee arthroplasty. J Arthroplasty 2016;31(7):1529–38.
2. Pelt CE, Grijalva R, Anderson L, et al. Two-Stage Revision TKA is associated with high complication and failure rates. Adv Orthop 2014;2014:659047.
3. Vince KG, Abdeen A. Wound problems in total knee arthroplasty. Clin Orthop Relat Res 2006; 452:88–90.
4. Qiu XS, Sun X, Chen DY, et al. Application of an articulating spacer in two-stage revision for severe infection after total knee arthroplasty. Orthop Surg 2010;2(4):299–304.
5. Gillespie BM, Thalib L, Ellwood D, et al. Effect of negative pressure wound therapy on wound complications in obese women after caesarean birth: a systematic review and meta-analysis. BJOG 2021;129(2):196–207.
6. Chang CC, Tang WR, Huang WL, et al. ASO visual abstract: algorithmic approach with negative pressure wound therapy improved survival in patients with synchronous hypopharyngeal and esophageal cancer undergoing pharyngolaryngoesophagectomy with gastric tube reconstruction. Ann Surg Oncol 2021;28(13):8996–9007.
7. Ayuso SA, Elhage SA, Okorji LM, et al. Closed-incision negative pressure therapy decreases wound morbidity in open abdominal wall reconstruction with concomitant panniculectomy. Ann Plast Surg 2021;88(4):429–33.
8. Ailaney N, Johns WL, Golladay GJ, et al. Closed incision negative pressure wound therapy for elective hip and knee arthroplasty: a systematic review and meta-analysis of randomized controlled trials. J Arthroplasty 2021;36(7):2402–11.
9. Newman JM, Siqueira MBP, Klika AK, et al. Use of closed incisional negative pressure wound therapy after revision total hip and knee arthroplasty in patients at high risk for infection: a prospective, randomized clinical trial. J Arthroplasty 2019;34(3): 554–9.e1.
10. Pagani NR, Moverman MA, Puzzitiello RN, et al. The cost-effectiveness of closed incisional negative pressure wound therapy for infection prevention after revision total knee arthroplasty. J Knee Surg 2021. https://doi.org/10.1055/s-0041-1724137.
11. Yaghmour KM, Hossain FS, Konan S. clinical and health-care cost analysis of negative pressure dressing in primary and revisiontotal knee arthroplasty: a systematic review and meta-analysis. J Bone Joint Surg Am 2020;541–8. Publish Ahead of Print.
12. Younger AS, Duncan CP, Masri BA. Surgical exposures in revision total knee arthroplasty. J Am Acad Orthop Surg 1998;6(1):55–64.
13. Della Valle CJ, Berger RA, Rosenberg AG. Surgical exposures in revision total knee arthroplasty. Clin Orthop Relat Res 2006;446:59–68.
14. Laskin RS. Ten steps to an easier revision total knee arthroplasty. J Arthroplasty 2002;17(4 Suppl 1): 78–82.
15. Mahomed N, McKee N, Solomon P, et al. Soft-tissue expansion before total knee arthroplasty in arthrodesed joints. A report of two cases. J Bone Joint Surg Br 1994;76(1):88–90.
16. Piuzzi NS, Costantini J, Carbo L, et al. Soft-tissue expansion beforetotal knee arthroplasty:a report of two cases. J Orthop Case Rep 2018;8(4):20–4.
17. Long WJ, Wilson CH, Scott SM, et al. 15-year experience with soft tissue expansion in total knee arthroplasty. J Arthroplasty 2012;27(3):362–7.
18. Osei DA, Rebehn KA, Boyer MI. Soft-tissue defects after total knee arthroplasty: management and

reconstruction. J Am Acad Orthop Surg 2016; 24(11):769–79.

19. Coombs DM, Churchill J, Cartwright P, et al. Soft tissue reconstruction for deep defects over a complicated total knee arthroplasty: a systematic review. J Knee Surg 2020;33(7):732–44.

20. Theil C, Stock ME, Gosheger G, et al. Gastrocnemius muscle flaps for soft tissue coverage in periprosthetic knee joint infection. J Arthroplasty 2020;35(12):3730–6.

21. Tetreault MW, Della Valle CJ, Bohl DD, et al. What factors influence the success of medial gastrocnemius flaps in the treatment of infected TKAs? Clin Orthop Relat Res 2016;474(3):752–63.

22. Warren SI, Murtaugh TS, Lakra A, et al. Treatment of periprosthetic knee infection with concurrent rotational muscle flap coverage is associated with high failure rates. J Arthroplasty 2018;33(10):3263–7.

23. Houdek MT, Wagner ER, Wyles CC, et al. Long-term outcomes of pedicled gastrocnemius flaps in total knee arthroplasty. J Bone Joint Surg Am 2018;100(10):850–6.

24. Auregan JC, Bégué T, Tomeno B, et al. Distally-based vastus lateralis muscle flap: a salvage alternative to address complex soft tissue defects around the knee. Orthop Traumatol Surg Res 2010;96(2):180–4.

25. Whiteside LA. Surgical technique: vastus medialis and vastus lateralis as flap transfer for knee extensor mechanism deficiency. Clin Orthop Relat Res 2013;471(1):221–30.

26. De Lorenzi F, Borelli F, Sala P, et al. Multistage latissimus dorsi flap with implant for complex postmastectomy reconstruction: an old but still current technique. Breast Care (Basel) 2021;16(4):396–401.

27. Hierner R, Reynders-Frederix P, Bellemans J, et al. Free myocutaneous latissimus dorsi flap transfer in total knee arthroplasty. J Plast Reconstr Aesthet Surg 2009;62(12):1692–700.

28. Raymond AC, Liddle AD, Alvand A, et al. Clinical outcome of free latissimus dorsi flaps for coverage of soft tissue defects in multiply revised total knee arthroplasties. J Arthroplasty 2021;36(2):664–9.

29. Casey WJ, Rebecca AM, Krochmal DJ, et al. Prophylactic flap reconstruction of the knee prior to total knee arthroplasty in high-risk patients. Ann Plast Surg 2011;66(4):381–7.

30. Azoury SC, Stranix JT, Piper M, et al. Attributes of perforator flaps for prophylatic soft tissue augmentation prior to definitive total knee arthroplasty. J Reconstr Microsurg 2021;37(1):51–8.

Management of Extensor Mechanism Disruption After Total Knee Arthroplasty

Michael R. Bisogno, MD, MBA*, Giles R. Scuderi, MD

KEYWORDS

- Extensor mechanism • Total knee arthroplasty • Patella tendon rupture
- Quadriceps tendon rupture

KEY POINTS

- Extensor mechanism disruptions following total knee arthroplasty are devastating injuries that are difficult to treat, with complication rates following surgical intervention ranging from 25% to 45%.
- Primary repair with and without augmentation is appropriate in acute injuries when adequate tissue and bone are available.
- Numerous reconstructive procedures have been described using autograft, allograft, and synthetic materials.
- Chronic extensor mechanism disruptions should be reconstructed with either an allograft or a synthetic mesh graft.
- Evaluation of preexisting components for malrotation and instability should be addressed before proceeding with an extensor mechanism repair or reconstruction.

INTRODUCTION

The extensor mechanism (EM) of the knee is a critical structure for ambulation and can experience 3 to 7 times the patient's body weight during stair climbing and squatting, respectively.[1] EM ruptures, of either the quadriceps tendon (QT) or patella tendon (PT), are a devastating complication in total knee arthroplasty (TKA). The incidence ranges from 0.17% to 1.4%,[2,3] with revision TKA increasing that risk.[4] Both the high failure and reoperation rate of PT ruptures may be due do the poor soft tissue coverage and the poor blood supply in the area.[5] Although a single traumatic event, such as a fall on a flexed knee, may result in a rupture of the EM, systemic diseases such as rheumatoid arthritis, diabetes mellitus, chronic renal failure, obesity, and hyperthyroidism may be predisposing factors.[1–3,6] Iatrogenic injury at the time of the initial TKA can also cause EM disruption,

especially when trying to gain exposure to a knee with limited range of motion or in the case of patella baja. Other local factors include a multioperated knee, multiple steroid injections, overresection of the patella, a lateral retinacular release that extends proximally and across the tendinous insertion of the vastus lateralis, patellectomy, and component malposition or malalignment. EM ruptures that occur within the first few weeks after surgery are likely related to errors in surgical technique.

PATIENT EVALUATION

Diagnosis of an EM rupture is easy when there are findings of an extensor lag and a palpable defect over either the quadriceps tendon or the patella tendon. A lateral radiograph may show a change in patella height compared with prior radiographs. Although a quadriceps tendon rupture may reveal patella infera

---

Orthopaedic Institute at Northwell Health, 210 East 64th Street, 4th Floor, New York, NY 10065, USA
* Corresponding author.
E-mail address: MBisogno@northwell.edu

Orthop Clin N Am 53 (2022) 277–286
https://doi.org/10.1016/j.ocl.2022.02.003

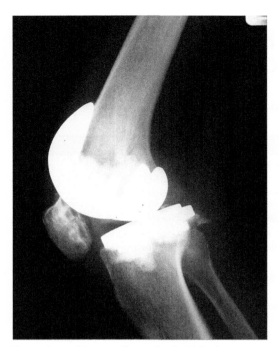

Fig. 1. Lateral knee radiograph of a TKA showing patella baja resulting from a QT rupture.

(Fig. 1), a patella tendon rupture may reveal a patella alta (Fig. 2). Beyond the simple diagnosis, it is important to assess the patient for factors that contribute to EM disruption. A history and physical examination should be taken to elicit symptoms and signs of patellar maltracking or instability, as these may have contributed to EM rupture.[6] If component malposition is suspected as a contributing cause for EM rupture, complete radiographic review or computed tomography scan should be performed[3]; this is important, as case series have reported approximately 80% of knees undergoing EM reconstruction require simultaneous component revision.[3]

TREATMENT OPTIONS

The timing, extent, and location of the injury to the EM will affect the treatment option (Fig. 3). Acute partial or incomplete injuries may be treated nonoperatively with brace or cast immobilization in extension for several weeks followed by gradual, controlled range of motion for several weeks thereafter. Several surgical techniques have been described for repair or reconstruction of the EM, although none are considered a gold standard. Reconstruction options include direct repair, repair with autogenous tissue, allograft reconstruction, and repair with synthetic grafts.

Although most complete EM disruptions require reconstruction, there are a few situations in which a nonoperative approach may be considered, primarily in a patient with comorbidities that preclude surgery or in an elderly, sedentary patient.[3,7] These patients will depend on a knee brace and walking aid for ambulation. Acute QT ruptures with an extension lag of less than 20° have an 85% success rate when immobilized in extension, as compared with a 75% success rate with operative intervention.[4,5] PT ruptures with an extension lag of less than 30° may also be considered for nonoperative treatment and immobilized in extension.[5] Nonoperative treatment is not appropriate for an active patient.

Primary repair of an EM disruption is indicated in acute injuries with adequate tissue and patella bone stock. An acute QT rupture with an extensor lag of more than 20° should be repaired.[4] These injuries may be treated primarily with either end-to-end repair, sutures through bone tunnels, or with the use of suture anchors.[8] However, a complication rate of 42% and 60% of patients reporting an unsatisfactory outcome after primary repair in the setting of a TKA suggests augmenting the graft is prudent.[4] A semitendinosus autograft is a common choice for augmentation.[4] Primary repair of PT ruptures has very poor outcomes[5]; this is believed to be from a high stress concentration, poor soft tissue coverage, a poor blood supply from repeated

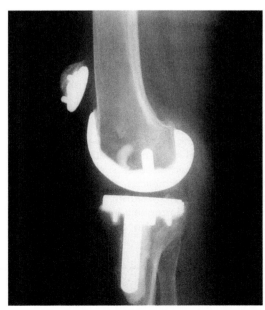

Fig. 2. Lateral knee radiograph of a TKA showing patella alta resulting from a PT rupture.

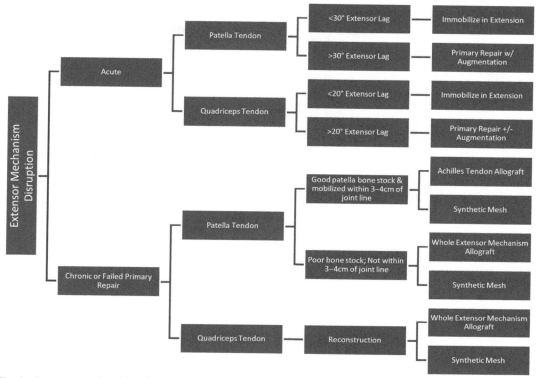

Fig. 3. A treatment algorithm for extensor mechanism disruptions in the setting of a TKA.

arthrotomies, and potentially malaligned components placing further stress on the repair.[5]

Reconstruction of the EM is the mainstay of treatment of EM disruptions. Several options exist for performing the reconstruction, including autograft, allograft, and synthetic grafts. Achilles tendon and complete EM allografts are commonly used, with the former appropriate for cases with an intact patella near the joint line.[3] A complete EM allograft is useful in the setting of a deficient patella, poor quality of the native EM tissue, or the inability to mobilize the patella to within 3 to 4 cm of the joint line.[3,4] Chronic EM ruptures require reconstruction, as primary repair has unacceptably high failure rates.[4] Chronic QT ruptures are most commonly augmented with a semitendinosus autograft.[4] An Achilles tendon allograft may be used for both QT and PT ruptures.[4] Other options for chronic QT ruptures include augmenting with autologous vastus medialis, lateralis, or medial head of the gastrocnemius, although there is less extensor lag when using the medial head of the gastrocnemius compared with advancing the vastus medialis and lateralis.[5] A medial gastrocnemius flap is required if there is significant proximal tibia bone loss, such that

the other allografts cannot be used, or in cases requiring soft tissue coverage over the anterior aspect of the knee.[4] This flap is often reserved for patients with prior infections, inadequate soft tissue coverage, or in cases of failed EM allografts.[9]

Synthetic mesh grafts have numerous benefits over allografts and autografts. Mesh has a decreased overall cost, no supply constraints, and no risk of disease transmission.[7] Further, the immediate strength from the mesh augments the repair, maintaining tensile strength without elongating, as well as acting as a scaffold for tissue ingrowth.[7] Histologic analysis of previously implanted mesh has shown excellent fibrous tissue infiltration without significant inflammation.[10]

SURGICAL TECHNIQUES

Prepare and drape the operative leg as usual for a TKA. A tourniquet is recommended, although a sterile tourniquet may be preferred for shorter thighs to allow for removal if necessary. The prior surgical incision is used, which is generally a midline skin incision. Full-thickness flaps are raised medially and laterally to expose the EM.

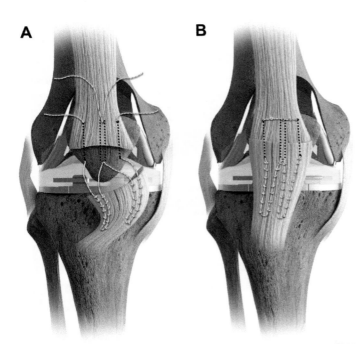

Fig. 4. Patella tendon repair showing Krackow stitches in the distal patella tendon passed through 3 bone tunnels through the patella (A). The sutures are then tied together while traction is maintained on the EM distally and patella tendon proximally (B).

PRIMARY REPAIR OF A PATELLA TENDON DISRUPTION WITH SEMITENDINOSUS AUGMENTATION

After full-thickness flaps are raised medially and laterally, debride the ends of the ruptured PT for direct repair. Run a nonabsorbable suture with a Krackow stitch along both the medial and lateral border of the PT. With a rupture of the PT from the inferior pole of the patella, drill bone tunnels through the patella and pass the nonabsorbable sutures through these holes (Fig. 4A). With the knee in full extension, tie the passed sutures together on the proximal aspect of the patella (Fig. 4B). Alternatively, suture anchors can be used in place of bone tunnels, particularly if there is inadequate patella bone stock remaining.[11] Ensure the medial and lateral retinaculum is repaired as needed. In the case of an avulsion of the patella tendon from the tibial tubercle, a Krackow stitch is run along the medial and lateral border of the PT, which are secured through a transosseous tunnel in the tibial tubercle. The repairs of avulsions from the tibial tubercle usually require augmentation with autogenous tissue.

This repair can be augmented with a semitendinosus autograft as described by Cadambi and Engh.[12] Extend the incision distally to expose the pes anserinus. Identify and harvest the semitendinosus, leaving it attached to its insertion along the medial tibia. Weave the tendon through the distal aspect of the QT from medial to lateral (Fig. 5). Finally, secure the free end of the tendon to itself near its insertion with #5 nonabsorbable sutures.

PRIMARY REPAIR OF A QUADRICEPS TENDON DISRUPTION

After full-thickness flaps are raised medially and laterally, as these ruptures are usually at the proximal pole of the patella, debride the ends of the ruptured QT for direct repair. Run a nonabsorbable stitch in a Krackow fashion through the remaining QT. Drill bone tunnels through the patella and pass the sutures through these holes (Fig. 6A). With the knee in full extension, tie the passed sutures together on the distal aspect of the patella (Fig. 6B). Alternatively, suture anchors can be used in place of bone tunnels, particularly if there is inadequate patella bone stock remaining.[11]

COMPLETE EXTENSOR MECHANISM ALLOGRAFT

After full-thickness flaps are raised medially and laterally, a midline incision is made through the existing EM from the QT to the tibial tubercle, excising any remaining patella. Medial and

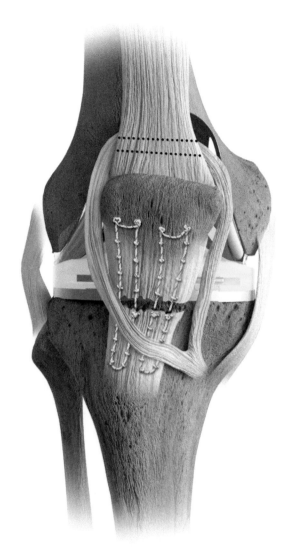

proximal edge at a 45° angle from the proximal insertion of the PT going proximally and posteriorly; this will form a dovetail joint with the host tibia. Finally, run two #5 nonabsorbable sutures along the medial and lateral aspects of the allograft QT in a locking Krackow fashion with the ends exiting proximally.[13]

Outline the graft tibial bone on the patient's tibia, paying close attention to the proximal location, as this will determine the patella height relative to the native joint. The patella should align with the top of the trochlea to allow for proper tracking. Cut the outline of the graft out, leaving the graft 1 mm wider than the trough for a more secure fit. Bevel the trough proximally to match that of the graft (**Fig. 7**A).[13]

Drill 2 to 3 holes in the tibia deep to the trough from medial to lateral and pass a stainless steel wire through each hole. Gently tamp the graft into the trough, dovetail first, with an up-and-in motion. Tighten the wires around the graft with the twisted part of the wire under the muscle on the lateral side of the tibia (**Fig. 7**B). Optionally, a cancellous screw with a washer may also be used to hold the graft in place, being careful not to fracture the graft bone.[13]

With the knee in full extension, pull the host QT distally with a stay suture. Pull the 2 previously placed sutures from the allograft QT proximally and pass through the proximal host QT. Although tension is maintained on both the host and graft tissue, tie these sutures together to hold in place. Continue suturing the graft to the more superficial medial and lateral flaps of the host QT while maintaining distal tension on the host QT. Once complete, suture the flaps together (**Fig. 7**C). Close the wound in layers, maintaining extension during the rest of the operation. Following wound closure, the knee is placed in a brace locked in extension for 8 to 12 weeks, followed by gradual and controlled range of motion in the ensuing weeks, and the patient is allowed to be weight-bearing as tolerated.[13]

Fig. 5. Patella tendon repair augmented with a semitendinosus autograft. The graft is passed through the proximal QT and sutured back onto itself.

lateral flaps of the entire EM should be raised.[13] At this point, the existing implant should be evaluated for malrotation and instability. If either is found, the components should be revised before moving forward. If using a stemmed tibial component, wires can be passed posterior to the stem, through the tibial bone for additional fixation of the graft.[13]

Prepare the allograft by cutting the allograft tibial tubercle along the sides of the PT, approximately 6 to 8 cm long. Then cut the tubercle 1 cm proximal to the PT insertion and just distal to the PT insertion. Taper the depth from 1.5 cm proximally to 1 cm distally. Next, bevel the

ACHILLES TENDON ALLOGRAFT

An Achilles tendon allograft with calcaneal bone may be used in situations where the patella bone stock is adequate and able to be mobilized to within 3 to 4 cm of the joint line.[4] The calcaneal bone is secured in a bone trough created in the tibial tubercle with either cerclage wires or screw fixation. The Achilles tendon is then divided into 3 arms in the shape of a trident. With the knee in full extension and the patella pulled distally, the

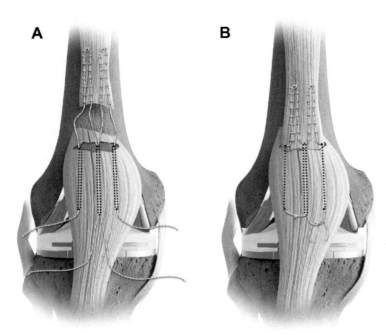

Fig. 6. Quadriceps tendon repair showing Krackow sutures in the QT passed through 3 bone tunnels through the patella (*A*). The sutures are then tied together while traction is maintained on the QT distally and remaining EM proximally (*B*).

central arm is secured to the injured patella tendon with nonabsorbable sutures. The medial and lateral arms are weaved through the medial and lateral retinaculum anchored into the quadriceps tendon at the superior pole of the patella with nonabsorbable sutures. The subcutaneous tissue is then closed over the allograft tissue. Following wound closure, the knee is

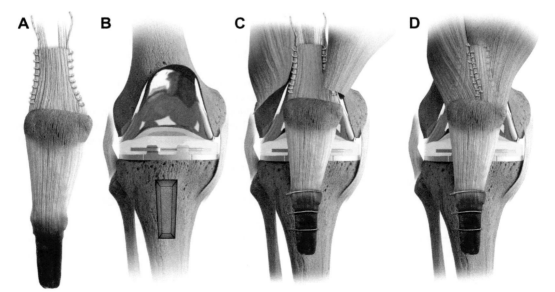

Fig. 7. Complete extensor mechanism allograft reconstruction (*A*). A bone trough is created in the host tibial tubercle (*B*). The graft is held in place in the tibia by stainless steel cerclage wires placed through the host tibial bone (*C*). The sutures from the graft are passed through the proximal QT and tied together, and the vastus medialis and vastus lateralis are closed over the graft and secured to it with nonabsorbable sutures (*D*).

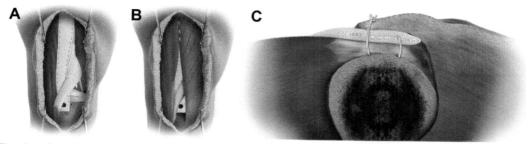

Fig. 8. Polypropylene mesh repair showing the tubularized mesh cemented and anchored into the tibial bone trough just distal to the tibial tray. The mesh is passed from deep to superficial on the lateral side of the patella tendon (A). The mesh is secured superficially to the medial edge of the vastus lateralis with traction on both the mesh and remaining EM (B). The vastus medialis is advanced and sutured in place over the mesh (C).

immobilized in full extension for 8 to 12 weeks, followed by gradual and controlled range of motion in the ensuing weeks.

POLYPROPYLENE MESH FOR AN EXTENSOR MECHANISM DISRUPTION

After full-thickness flaps are raised medially and laterally, bluntly mobilize the vastus medialis and vastus lateralis for maximal EM excursion.[13] At this point, the existing implant should be evaluated for malrotation and instability. If either is found, the components should be revised.[13]

Prepare the synthetic nonabsorbable mesh by rolling a single sheet (25 cm × 35.5 cm) over itself to form a 2- to 2.5-cm wide tube and hold in place with a running #5 nonabsorbable suture along the free edge. The mesh can be secured intramedullary in the tibia during cementation of the tibial component if it is being revised. Use a burr to create a trough for the mesh to exist just below the anteromedial aspect of the tibial tray. Insert the mesh at least a few centimeters into the tibial canal. Cement in place and secure further with a screw and washer, taking care to aim away from the tibial keel or stem.[13]

After the components are revised as needed and the mesh is secured, free a layer of fat pad or synovial tissue to pass between the tibial tray and mesh; this will prevent damage to the mesh from rubbing against the tibial tray. Attach this tissue layer to the mesh with a nonabsorbable suture. Incise a vertical slit on the lateral aspect of the PT to pass the mesh from deep to superficial, laying the mesh on top of the vastus lateralis (Fig. 8A). With the knee in full extension, align the medial edges of the mesh and vastus lateralis, pulling tension on the vastus distally and graft proximally. Secure in place with #5 nonabsorbable sutures (Fig. 8B). Extensively advance the vastus medialis on top of the mesh so that it is completely covered by host

tissue.[10] Suture in place under tension with additional #5 nonabsorbable sutures (Fig. 8C). The wound is closed in layers, maintaining extension during the rest of the operation. Following wound closure, the knee is immobilized in full extension for 8 to 12 weeks, and the patient is allowed to be weight-bearing as tolerated.[13]

If the EM reconstruction is being performed along with revision of the components, the mesh can be placed in the tibial canal just before the tibial component placement and ultimately secured when the tibia is cemented in place. The reconstruction then commences as detailed earlier (Fig. 9).

KEY SURGICAL POINTS

Allografts should be fresh frozen as opposed to freeze-dried.[6] Further, irradiated grafts have a higher complication rate and thus should be avoided.[7] Complete EM allografts should match the laterality of the operative extremity.[6] The tibial bone stock of complete EM grafts should be at least 5 cm, and the QT should be no shorter than 5 cm.[6]

Regardless of the repair or reconstruction method chosen, the knee must be in full extension during tensioning[4]; this must be maintained throughout the closure. Postoperatively, it is critical to immobilize the extremity in full extension, either with a cast or a brace for an extended period of time, up to 8 to 12 weeks, followed by gradual and controlled range of motion in the ensuing weeks. During the period of immobilization, a brace is preferred for wound inspection if the patient is felt to be reliable.

DISCUSSION

Overall, extension lag of greater than 30° was the most common complication in EM repair or reconstruction, occurring in 45% of patients.[1]

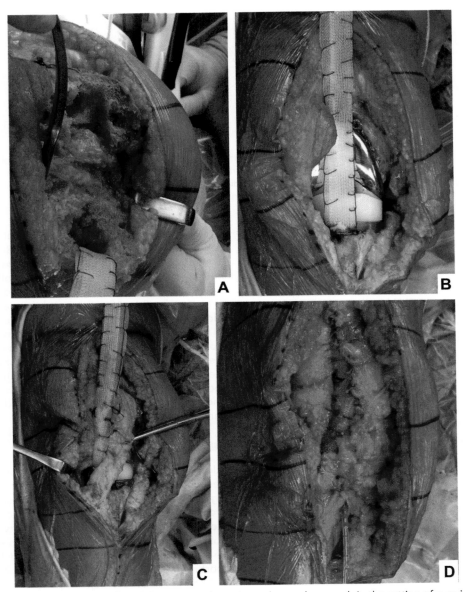

Fig. 9. Intraoperative photos of an EM reconstruction using polypropylene mesh in the setting of a revision TKA. The mesh is placed in the tibial canal before tibial component cementation (*A*). The revision components are cemented in place, securing the mesh in the tibial canal (*B*). The mesh is passed from deep to superficial on the lateral side of the patella tendon (*C*). The mesh is then secured superficially to the medial edge of the vastus lateralis. The vastus medialis is advanced and sutured over the mesh (*D*).

Rerupture and infection were also common, at 25% and 23%, respectively.[1] Contracture was much more rare at 3%.[1] Surgery within 2 weeks of injury was found to be a significant factor for better outcomes; poor outcomes occurred in 15% of cases treated surgically within 2 weeks of injury as compared with 45% of cases treated after 2 weeks.[14] A history of a prosthetic joint infection was an independent risk factor for

poor outcomes, with an odds ratio (OR) of 4.6.[14]

For QT repairs, a small study of 7 patients found that primary repair provided good functional outcome at 3 months for partial ruptures and 6 months for complete ruptures.[2] The cause of failure in this series was most commonly sudden overloading of the QT leading to mechanical failure.[2] Other studies have reported reoperation rates up to 35% and prosthetic joint infection at 12%.[2]

Primary repair of patellar tendon ruptures without augmentation often results in unsatisfactory results.[3] Compared with the complication rate of 25% after QT repairs, Vajapey found a significantly higher complication rate of 63% in PT repairs.[1] However, reconstruction of the PT, which included autografts, allografts, and mesh, was found to be significantly improved with a complication rate of 26%[1]; this was also noted by Courtney who reported that direct repair of PT ruptures was an independent risk factor for poor outcomes as compared with QT repairs (OR 10.6, 95% confidence interval 1.7–64.4, $P = .011$).[14]

Allograft reconstruction was historically the preferred method for EM repairs, although immune reactions and structural changes in the tissues lead to late extensor lag.[5,7] In a series of 16 allograft reconstructions for a variety of reasons (1 acute QT rupture, 8 chronic PT ruptures, 5 failed PT repairs, and 2 failed QT repairs), the mean extension lag was reduced from $35° \pm 16°$ preoperatively to $14° \pm 18°$ ($P < .001$) at final follow-up.[9]

However, allografts have a high cost and relatively high risk of infection. Vyas showed that of 8 failed allograft reconstructions that were reoperated with another allograft, all failed to improve, and 25% of the patients developed infections.[5] In these failed scenarios, especially with a prosthetic infection, salvage procedures such as fusions or amputations may need to be considered.

The use of synthetic materials such as Marlex Mesh (BD, Franklin Lakes, NJ, USA) has shown promising results. Browne and Hanssen reported using mesh in 13 patients for PT reconstruction.[3] Five patients underwent primary reconstruction, and all had a significant improvement in extensor lag at an average of 42 months.[3] Of the 7 patients who failed an EM reconstruction with allograft, 3 succeeded but 3 failed again and 1 developed an infection requiring an arthrodesis.[3] No late extensor lag was observed during the follow-up period.[3] Two studies, one by Deren and the other by Shau, both found a comparable failure rate of 25% for both mesh and allografts, with no differences between outcomes and infections.[15,16] A meta-analysis also found no significant difference in success rates between synthetic mesh (78%) and allografts (73%).[16] One case series showed 9 of 13 reconstructions with synthetic mesh had less than 10° of extensor lag without progression.[4] Of the remaining 4, 3 failed and 1 had a recurrent infection.[4] A larger study of 77 patients showed 84% had successful results at 4-year follow-up.[4] From a resource utilization standpoint, synthetic materials are approximately 50 times less expensive than allografts and much easier logistically to handle and store.[7]

SUMMARY

EM disruptions in the setting of a prior TKA are potentially devastating injuries. Exclusive primary repair is indicated in only a few limited settings, with reconstruction being the mainstay of treatment. Following the treatment algorithm appropriately increases the likelihood of satisfactory outcomes; however, patients must be counseled on the high complication rates of these procedures.

CLINICS CARE POINTS

- Evaluation of preexisting components for malposition or malrotation and instability is critical and should be addressed before proceeding with an EM repair or reconstruction.

- Consider nonoperative treatment in patients who are poor surgical candidates for an extensive reconstruction.

- PT primary repairs are an option for acute ruptures with adequate tissue and patella bone stock and may be augmented with either autograft, allograft, or a synthetic graft to avoid high complication rates.

- Allografts should be fresh frozen and nonirradiated for improved mechanical properties.

- Complete EM allografts should match the laterality of the operative extremity. There is no need to resurface the patella.

- Synthetic mesh grafts are a promising and inexpensive option for EM reconstructions, with data generally supporting at least equivalent to complete EM allografts.

- Repairs and reconstructions of the EM must be done with the knee in full extension and with tension held on both the distal and proximal ends of the EM. Do not flex the knee or test the repair or reconstruction.

- Ensure all allografts and synthetic grafts are completely covered by host tissues before skin closure to optimize healing.

- Immobilize patients postoperatively for 8 to 12 weeks in either a brace or a cast. A brace allows for easier wound care but requires a compliant patient.

DISCLOSURE

M.R. Bisogno: nothing to disclose. G.R. Scuderi: Royalties: Zimmer Biomet; Consultant: Zimmer Biomet; 3M KCI; Enhanced Medical Nutrition; Stock and stock options: ROM Tech; Force Therapeutics; Enhanced Medical Nutrition; Editorial Board: Journal of Knee Surgery; Book Royalties: Elsevier; Springer; Thieme; World Scientific.

REFERENCES

1. Vajapey SP, Blackwell RE, Maki AJ, et al. Treatment of Extensor Tendon Disruption After Total Knee Arthroplasty: A Systematic Review. J Arthroplasty 2019;34(6):1279–86.
2. Chhapan J, Sankineani SR, Chiranjeevi T, et al. Early quadriceps tendon rupture after primary total knee arthroplasty. Knee 2018;25(1):192–4.
3. Bates MD, Springer BD. Extensor mechanism disruption after total knee arthroplasty. J Am Acad Orthop Surg 2015;23(2):95–106.
4. Ng J, Balcells-Nolla P, James PJ, et al. Extensor mechanism failure in total knee arthroplasty. EFORT Open Rev 2021;6(3):181–8.
5. Vyas P, Cui Q. Management options for extensor mechanism discontinuity in patients with total knee arthroplasty. Cureus 2020. https://doi.org/10.7759/cureus.9225.
6. Sain A, Bansal H, Pattabiraman K, et al. Extensor mechanism reconstruction using allograft following total knee arthroplasty: a review of current practice. Cureus 2021;13(1):e12803.
7. Wood TJ, Leighton J, Backstein DJ, et al. Synthetic Graft Compared With Allograft Reconstruction for Extensor Mechanism Disruption in Total Knee Arthroplasty: A Multicenter Cohort Study. J Am Acad Orthop Surg 2019;27(12):451–7.
8. Heer ST, O'Dowd J, Butler RR, et al. Quadriceps Tendon Rupture Following Total Knee Arthroplasty. Open Orthop J 2019;13(1):250–4.
9. Lim CT, Amanatullah DF, Huddleston JI, et al. Reconstruction of Disrupted Extensor Mechanism After Total Knee Arthroplasty. J Arthroplasty 2017;32(10):3134–40.
10. Cohen-Rosenblum A, Volaric A, Browne JA. Retrieval analysis of a failed synthetic mesh extensor mechanism reconstruction after total knee arthroplasty. Arthroplasty Today 2018;4(4):447–51.
11. Parker DA, Dunbar MJ, Rorabeck CH. Extensor mechanism failure associated with total knee arthroplasty: prevention and management. J Am Acad Orthop Surg 2003;11(4):238–47.
12. Cadambi A, Engh GA. Use of a semitendinosus tendon autogenous graft for rupture of the patellar ligament after total knee arthroplasty. A report of seven cases. J Bone Joint Surg Am 1992;74(7):974–9.
13. Tria AJ, Scuderi GR, Cushner FD, et al. Complex cases in total knee arthroplasty : a compendium of current techniques. 1st edition. Cham, Switzerland: Springer International Publishing : Imprint: Springer; 2018.
14. Courtney PM, Edmiston TA, Pflederer CT, et al. Is There Any Role for Direct Repair of Extensor Mechanism Disruption Following Total Knee Arthroplasty? J Arthroplasty 2018;33(7):S244–8.
15. Shau D, Patton R, Patel S, et al. Synthetic mesh vs. allograft extensor mechanism reconstruction in total knee arthroplasty - A systematic review of the literature and meta-analysis. Knee 2018;25(1):2–7.
16. Deren ME, Pannu TS, Villa JM, et al. Meta-analysis comparing allograft to synthetic reconstruction for extensor mechanism disruption after total knee arthroplasty. J Knee Surg 2021;34(3):338–50.

Trauma

Lower Extremity Soft Tissue Reconstruction Review Article

Ahmed M. Mansour, MD[a,*], Aaron Jacobs, MD[a],
Mamtha S. Raj, MD, MA[a], Frank G. Lee, BSE[b],
Weston Terrasse, MD, MS[a], Sean J. Wallace, MD[c],
Nathan F. Miller, MD[a]

KEYWORDS

• Flap • Muscle • Orthoplastic • Reconstruction • Soft tissue • Lower Extremity

INTRODUCTION

Reconstruction plays a valuable role in the management of lower extremity wounds for limb salvage. The goals of reconstruction are to improve function and quality of life, return to work, and pain reduction while providing a long-lasting durable reconstruction.[1–3] The plastics and reconstructive surgical approach in conjunction with the orthopedic or trauma team, referred often as the "orthoplastic" approach, can yield the best outcomes for patients.[4,5] The following sections discuss reconstruction principles and techniques that can be applied broadly for lower extremity wounds secondary to trauma, infection, and tumor resection.

ORTHOPLASTIC APPROACH

A team approach between plastics and orthopedics can optimize surgical planning and thereby avail the patient to the best treatment plan. In orthoplastic cases, fracture stability and reduction precede soft tissue reconstruction. However, early involvement of the reconstructive and microsurgery teams at the index procedure can maximize available flap options by providing input on surgical decisions such as

location of incisions or placement of external fixation pins.[4] Successful high-volume centers in orthopedic and reconstructive trauma have created a culture and system that values a multidisciplinary approach; this involves not only the orthopedic and reconstructive surgical teams but also infectious disease, wound care, social work, and rehabilitation specialists.[5]

TYPES OF CASES

The types of cases that benefit from reconstruction are diverse and include, but are not limited to, high-velocity and off-road motorized vehicle accidents, open tibia-fibula fractures, degloving injuries, gunshot wounds, and combat-related wounds. The most common classification system for lower extremity wounds is the Gustilo system, which is based on extent of wound.[6] Gustilo type I and II involve less than 1 cm and 1 to 10 cm wounds, respectively. Gustilo type III are greater than 10 cm wounds and are further subdivided into A (adequate tissue coverage), B (wounds requiring soft tissue coverage), and C (wounds requiring vascular repair) (Table. 1). Gustilo types IIIB and IIIC are the predominate types indicated for reconstruction. Other classification systems exist such as the Tscherne

Conflict of Interest and Financial Disclosures: all of the authors listed above have no conflict of interest or financial disclosures.

[a] Division of Plastic and Reconstructive Surgery, Lehigh Valley Health Network, 1250 South Cedar Crest Boulevard, Allentown, PA 18103, USA; [b] University of South Florida Morsani College of Medicine, 2049 Street Wood Street, Allentown, PA 18103, USA; [c] Division of Plastic and Reconstructive Surgery, Lehigh Valley Health Network, 3701 Corriere Road, Suite 15, Easton, PA 18045, USA
* Corresponding author.
E-mail address: ahmed.mansour@lvhn.org

Table 1
Gustilo classification of open fractures

Gustilo Classification	Description
Type I	Open fracture with soft tissue wound <1 cm
Type II	Open fracture with soft tissue wound 1–10 cm
Type III A	Open fracture, >10 cm wound, extensive soft tissue injury, without periosteal stripping
Type III B	Open fracture, >10 cm wound, periosteal stripping present
Type III C	Open fracture with an associated vascular injury that requires repair for limb survival

classification and the OTA-OFC (Orthopedic Trauma Association—Open Fracture Classification); however, these are not universally used as the Gustilo system.[1]

LIMB SALVAGE VERSUS AMPUTATION

"Life before limb" is the basic tenet when considering limb salvage versus amputation. Once life-threatening injuries or sepsis can be safely ruled out, the initial evaluation of limb salvage and reconstruction must consider the long-term outlook.[7] The reconstructive surgeon is challenged with the question of "will limb salvage lead to meaningful long-term outcomes compared to amputation?" in terms of function, performance, mobility, and returning to work. Complications such as secondary amputation, osteomyelitis, flap failure, and nonunion must be considered.[1,2,8,9] The sentinel LEAP study showed no major difference in Sickness Index Profile between amputation and limb salvage and at 7-year follow-up, maintained no difference.[3,10] Follow-up studies to LEAP have been done, including the METALS and OUTLET studies.[11,12] The conclusion from the LEAP study demonstrated reconstruction and limb salvage was noninferior to amputation; this led to increased utilization of reconstruction.

If amputation is the ultimate decision, consultation from the plastic surgery team can still be beneficial. Free tissue techniques such as transferring the fillet of the heel sole to the stump can provide more durability and wear resistance for prosthetic fitting.[13,14] Other beneficial techniques plastic surgeons can offer at the time of amputations include targeted muscle reinnervation and regenerative peripheral nerve interface to help reduce incidence of phantom limb pain and maintain muscle bulk at the amputation stump.[15]

RECONSTRUCTION LADDER

If limb salvage and reconstruction has been decided, the type of approach must be chosen next. A popular paradigm is "the reconstruction ladder," which favors the simplest solution first and resorting to more complex, intensive solutions only if the simpler approach fails or not feasible.[8,9] The ladder generally follows the order of healing by secondary intention, primary closure, skin graft, local tissue rearrangement flaps, distant pedicled flaps, and free flap transfer. A more recent paradigm shift to the reconstruction ladder has been proposed, termed "the reconstruction elevator," which aims to use the best long-term solution for a given problem irrespective of the complexity.[1,2,16]

TIMING

Timing for lower extremity reconstruction is important, and recognizing emergent indications is necessary. Furthermore, an understanding of timing of the healing process with respect to inflammation, fibrosis, and scarring will give the plastic surgeon an advantage in reconstruction and flap success.[17] Originally, the golden window established by Godina in 1986 for reconstruction was 3 days.[18] A study by Lee and colleagues provided evidence that supported extending the timing window to 10 days.[19] An analysis showed significantly fewer flap failure rates in the less than 10 day group versus greater than or equal to 10 days; however, the study did not measure other complication endpoints such as nonunion, infection, osteomyelitis, and amputations.[19] This study gave credence to what experienced surgeons anecdotally recognized; successful reconstruction can exceed the Godina's "3-day rule." An explanation for the increase in timing has been attributed to the advent of negative pressure wound therapy, which temporizes the wound by improving local fluid management and edema, while allowing granulation tissue formation before definitive coverage.[20] However, earlier soft tissue coverage is typically required in the setting of exposed critical structures such as bone, vessel, hardware, joint, tendon, and nerve. Generally, desiccation poses risks of arterial rupture or permanent nerve damage, and prolonged duration of exposed orthopedic implants significantly increases infection risk.[17]

WOUND PREPARATION

Soft tissue debridement and clearing devitalized tissue is the cornerstone of lower extremity reconstruction. Dead tissue is a nidus for infection and, if not treated correctly, requires multiple reoperations and may lead to amputation. Therefore, surgical debridement is paramount for infection prevention. Quantitative cultures can be ordered to assess degree of contamination with a threshold of greater than 10^5 bacteria/gram of tissue; however, burns are an exception.[17] Systemic antibiotics are warranted in osteomyelitis, and consult to infectious disease may be warranted to manage appropriate antibiotics based on culture data. Antibiotic impregnated cement beads or spacers can be used for dead space management (in areas where unwanted blood, fluid, and bacteria fill empty spaces). Beads are ideal for short-term use and offer more surface area for antibiotic elution; however, they can become affixed in granulation tissue and biofilm. Spacers are suitable for long-term use because of the membrane that often forms and can be useful in later reconstructive efforts. Irrigation is a useful tool; however, it should not precede or replace sharp surgical debridement. Irrigation with gravity lavage is preferred to high pressure, as high pressure can cause further tissue damage and drive contaminants into tissue.[21]

PRINCIPLES OF SOFT TISSUE COVERAGE

The principles of soft tissue coverage in traumatic lower extremity reconstruction ideally follow replacing missing tissue with tissue of similar characteristics (size, location, depth, complexity, function, and consistency).[1,4,8] The breadth of locoregional transfer techniques is extensive and includes V-Y, bipedicled, keystone, propeller, island, and paddle flaps. Generally, free tissue transfer and propeller are used in the distal third of the lower leg; however it is technically more challenging and requires microsurgery experience.[22]

Flap types include muscle only: myocutaneous (muscle with attached skin) and fasciocutaneous (fascia with attached skin). Traditionally, the vascularity supplied by muscle was thought to be optimal for fracture healing and osteomyelitis and ideal for obliterating cavities where bulk was needed.[2,17] It offered pressure

sensibility but lacked surface sensibility. When selecting muscle flaps for use, muscle groups that share functionality as gastrocnemius and soleus or rectus femoris and vastus lateralis can be harvested without significantly compromising function in their respective areas because of functional redundancy. The vasculature of a muscle flap is critical in harvesting. The Mathes and Nahai classification system delineates between a single dominant vessel (type 1) and a multiple/variegated blood supply (type 2–5) (Table 2).

Recently, a shift in favor of fasciocutaneous has begun to emerge.[23,24] Cho showed equivalent outcomes between muscle and fasciocutaneous free flaps in lower extremity traumatic reconstruction; however, fasciocutaneous flaps required longer operative times and had a steeper learning curve.[23]

LOWER EXTREMITY RECONSTRUCTION OPTIONS

Thigh Soft Tissue Reconstruction

The thigh offers considerable freedom in reconstruction options due to its large size, few compartments, and muscle groups that share similar movement and function. Because the thigh is a vascular region, use of skin grafts is possible (Fig. 1). Transferring local tissue by V-Y or bipedicled approaches can be readily performed. The decision to use an ipsilateral or contralateral donor region depends on availability. Using donor flap tissue from the ipsilateral thigh limits the reconstruction and surgical area to one side and protects the other leg's function for ambulation. However, using the contralateral thigh may be necessitated if the wound defect is substantially sizable or no options exist ipsilaterally. The most common local reconstruction options are rectus femoris, sartorius, gracilis,

Table 2	
Mathes and Nahai classification of muscle vascular supply	
Mathes & Nahai Classification	**Description**
Type I	One vascular pedicle
Type II	One dominant pedicle and minor pedicles
Type III	Two dominant pedicles
Type IV	Segmental vascular pedicles
Type V	One dominant pedicel and secondary segmental pedicles

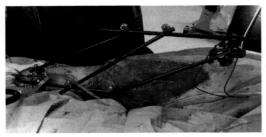

Fig. 1. A 32-year-old man after right femur ORIF after MVA with significant soft tissue loss of his medial thigh. The bulky, healthy musculature of the thigh allowed for successful skin graft take to heal his wound. MVA, motor vehicle accident; ORIF, open reduction and internal fixation.

vastus lateralis, tensor fascia lata, anterolateral thigh, and biceps femoris flaps. Free tissue transfer for thigh wounds is rarely used, given the local options readily available.

The sartorius is a long flap that can be modified for soft tissue coverage as needed. Used mainly by vascular surgeons for vascular graft coverage in the groin, the sartorius can be harvested without significant compromise to function. As a Mathes and Nahai type IV, the sartorius has segmental blood supply contributions from the superficial circumflex iliac artery, branches of the superficialis femoris and profunda femoris, and descending geniculate arteries (Fig. 2). Caution must be taken to preserve the segmental bloody supply and avoid vascular embarrassment.

The gracilis is a Mathes and Nahai type II flap that can be used as a muscle or myocutaneous flap. Its primary blood supply is the ascending branch of the medial circumflex femoral artery with contributing branches from the superficial femoral artery (see Fig. 2). It can be used as a

pedicled flap or free flap. If not deinnervated, it can maintain motor function via anterior branch of the obturator nerve.

The rectus femoris is a large local flap that can be adapted as muscle or myocutaneous as needed. It is a Mathes and Nahai type II flap with a descending branch of the lateral circumflex femoral artery dominant blood supply and minor pedicles from musculocutaneous perforators. Sensation can be maintained with an intact intermediate cutaneous nerve of the thigh (Fig. 3).

The vastus lateralis is a muscle or musculocutaneous flap that can offer bulk and coverage. It has Mathes and Nahai type I blood supply from the lateral circumflex femoral artery. The nerve supply runs along the pedicle and can provide voluntary control. It spans the entire length of the thigh between its origin at the greater trochanter and gluteal tuberosity to the distal insertion at the patella. The vastus lateralis, tensor fascia lata, and anterolateral thigh are chimeric flap options and offer similar coverage with differing tissue amount.

The tensor fascia lata is a Mathes and Nahai type I musculocutaneous flap for soft tissue coverage due to its ability to offer sizable coverage and easy of harvesting. The anatomic relationship is superficial to the vastus lateralis and lateral to the sartorius. The lateral femoral circumflex vessel pedicle arises at the proximal-middle thigh from the profunda femoris,

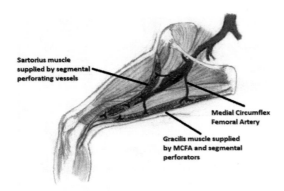

Fig. 2. Medial circumflex femoral artery (MCFA) supplying the gracilis and sartorius muscle.

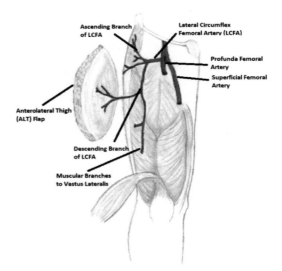

Fig. 3. The lateral circumflex femoral artery branches supplying the tensor fascia lata (TFL) muscle, anterolateral thigh (ALT) fasciocutaneous flap, and the vastus lateralis muscle.

providing a large arc of rotation that explains why it can be used in abdominal wall reconstruction. It can provide sensation via the lateral femoral cutaneous nerve and voluntary control via the descending branch of the superior gluteal nerve. The donor site can be closed primarily and has limited donor morbidity.

The anterolateral thigh flap is a fasciocutaneous flap with increasing versatility for coverage. Its location is similar to the vastus lateralis; however, it lacks the bulk of a muscle flap. Its blood supply is from the perforating branches of the descending branch of the lateral femoral circumflex that emerges between the rectus femoris and vastus lateralis muscles.

In the rare circumstances where local muscle or fasciocutaneous flap options are not available, the pedicled rectus abdominis muscular or myocutaneous flap can be used for large full-thickness defects in the proximal thigh, groin, or buttocks. These flaps follow a Mathes and Nahai type III arrangement with dual supply from the deep superior epigastric and deep inferior epigastric arteries. The general skin laxity and available tissue found in the abdominal tissue region gives ample large skin and bulk if needed.

LOWER LEG SOFT TISSUE RECONSTRUCTION

The focus here is on local soft tissue options and perforator flaps, which are not always possible depending on the extent and location of the wound; however, many options exist that may preclude the need for a free tissue transfer.[25] The lower leg is divided into thirds when defining reconstructive options (upper, middle, and lower).

Upper Third

The upper third is defined by the area immediately surrounding and including the knee.[9,25] Traditionally larger defects with periosteal stripping from the knee down require free flaps in order to sufficiently reconstruct the defect and achieve the goal of coverage and best functional outcome; however, there are options available for smaller defects.[25] The most commonly used flaps for knee or upper third defects of the lower leg include the gastrocnemius muscle and tibialis anterior muscle flaps.

The gastrocnemius muscle is composed of a lateral and medial head that are supplied by the lateral and medial sural arteries, respectively. Given the fact that there are 2 heads available, sacrificing one does not result in loss of this key function if the soleus remains functional. The medial head of the gastrocnemius is larger, provides a longer flap option, and generally preferred for coverage of knee defects.

Another option includes the anterior tibialis muscle; however, this is a much smaller muscle compared with the gastrocnemius and usually more useful for coverage of defects on the proximal anterior tibia. This muscle's blood supply is from multiple perforators from the anterior tibial artery. The anterior tibialis muscle is responsible for dorsiflexion of the foot and not as expendable as the gastrocnemius, given this important function.[9] Given this necessary function and segmental blood supply, the entire muscle is not normally sacrificed; the muscle can be used as a sagittal split muscle flap and is used to cover those proximal tibial defects, as well as some middle-third defects.[26]

Other options include propeller flaps from perforators of the 3 major vessels of the lower leg: the peroneal artery, anterior tibial artery, and posterior tibial artery.[25] These are great options for reconstruction when available, as they maintain underlying musculature, avoid damaging the source vessel, and avoid the need for microvascular anastomoses.[27] For the knee, there are also possible perforator flap options from the genicular system.[25] These are viable options that can be found using a handheld doppler or duplex ultrasound, identifying the most robust perforator adjacent to the defect that would be amenable for reconstruction. Other options for reconstruction include keystone island perforator flaps, described as a multiperforator curvilinear trapezoidal advancement flap adjacent to an elliptical defect.[28] All of these flaps are viable options for defects of the upper third depending on the surgeon's comfort level and magnitude of the wound at hand.

Middle Third

When considering the middle third and distal third of the leg, the same basic principles of the upper third remain; however, available options vary based on available tissue, blood supply, and muscles. The soleus muscle is a major workhouse flap for reconstruction of the middle third.[9] Proximally the muscle is supplied by branches from the popliteal artery, the medial muscle belly is supplied by posterior tibial artery branches, and the lateral muscle belly by peroneal artery perforators. The muscle can be disinserted and transposed over wounds on the middle third of the lower leg but requires ligation of those more distal perforators to allow for a greater arch of rotation. If the defect is small enough, a hemisoleus muscle flap may be performed.[9]

Other options for reconstruction in this area include the anterior tibialis, flexor digitorum longus, extensor digitorum longus, extensor digitorum hallucis, and longus. These options are limited for smaller defects of the lower leg and mostly only amenable for wounds on the lower portion of the middle third of the leg. Functional loss of the donor muscle may be seen, so care must be taken to either preserve the function or educate the patient on functional deficits that may be incurred from these reconstructive options.[29]

As with the upper third of the leg, perforator flaps are also viable options for reconstruction with the most robust perforators coming from the posterior tibial artery. The anterior tibial artery also provides perforators for fasciocutaneous flap options in the more proximal tibial defects. Lastly, medial sural artery perforator flaps can be based proximally or distally to provide necessary coverage for defects of the upper and middle lower leg.[27]

Lower Third

Traditionally the distal or lower third of the leg has not been amenable to many local reconstructive options, as there are not reliable local muscle flaps and thus free flaps were often recommended.[25] With increased understanding of vascularity, local fasciocutaneous flaps have been shown to be effective and great options for these tough defects.[9,29]

The distally based or "reverse" sural fasciocutaneous flap is also referred to as a neuro-skin flap due to the arterial supply coming from the median superficial sural artery that accompanies the sural nerve.[9,29] The pedicle is based on the retrograde flow through perforators from the peroneal artery to the superficial sural (see

"foot and ankle soft tissue reconstruction" section for more details).[29] A skin paddle with a diameter as large as 14 cm on the proximal posterior calf can be harvested with the flap and transposed into the wound.[9]

The propeller flap with unequal lengths of fasciocutaneous tissue on either side of the perforator provides multiple reconstructive options based on perforators from the major vessels of the lower extremity (**Fig. 4**).[29] The anterior tibial artery also gives off a cluster of distal perforators that can be used for coverage of even the lateral malleolus.[27] If all else fails or the patient is not a candidate for any of the aforementioned procedures and the patient is not a candidate for free tissue transfer, the cross-leg flap remains a viable and historical option for reconstructing a distal lower extremity wound.[29]

FOOT AND ANKLE SOFT TISSUE RECONSTRUCTION

Reconstruction of the foot and ankle soft tissue presents unique challenges to plastic surgeons, orthopedic surgeons, and podiatric surgeons alike.[1] One must consider the compressive forces of weight-bearing loads exerted on the foot and ankle region when evaluating patients for reconstruction. Moreover, a well-reconstructed foot must be able to both tolerate the sheering stress while bearing weight and contour well to accommodate wearing a shoe.[30]

GENERAL FOOT AND ANKLE RECONSTRUCTION

The foot can be divided into 7 distinct subunits based on aesthetic and reconstructive goals (**Fig. 5**). Subunit 1 encompasses the dorsal and volar aspects of all toes. Moderate aesthetic considerations must be taken with reconstruction. Free tissue transfer is usually required for reconstruction. Subunit 2 is the weight-bearing

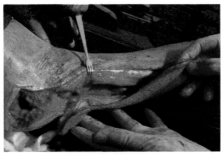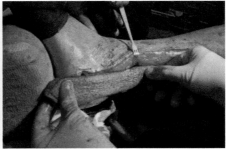

Fig. 4. A 63-year-old woman with a lateral calcaneal wound after diabetic wound debridement. A propeller flap based off a single peroneal perforator was harvested and rotated 180° for wound coverage.

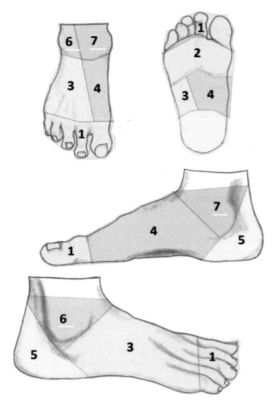

Fig. 5. Multiple views of the ankle and foot with 7 labeled aesthetic and functional divisions.

forefoot. This region has a high functional usage and requires a highly durable, yet pliable reconstruction. Subunits 3 and 4 encompass the dorsum of the foot with a lower function and high aesthetic demand. Again, thin and pliable coverage is needed. Subunit 5 is the weight-bearing heel and Achilles region. This region has a high functional demand and requires a durable and thicker kind of coverage. Subunits 6 and 7 are the lateral and medial malleoli, respectively. These regions need to be thin but, most of all, pliable to allow for good ankle movement.[31] Later the authors discuss the reconstructive options for these subunits.

RECONSTRUCTION OF THE PLANTAR FOOT

Skin grafting to the plantar aspect of the foot has been one accepted method of soft tissue reconstruction. For superficial defects where no bone, tendon without paratenon, or hardware is exposed, a split-thickness skin graft may be considered. Glabrous skin for grafting was noted to be superior to nonglabrous skin, as the risks

of hyperkeratotic deposition at the skin graft margins and contracture were less.[30] Full-thickness skin grafting is another option for reconstruction. Typically harvested from the medial instep or from the avulsed tissue in the setting of trauma, full-thickness skin grafts were found to have an 81% of take to the wound bed.[30]

Dermal substitutes may also be considered before skin grafting to add bulk to the wound and help with creation of a proper wound bed for future skin grafting. Integra, Apligraf (Organogenesis Inc, Canton, MA, USA), and acellular dermal matrix (Musculoskeletal Transplant Foundation, Edison, NJ, USA).[30]

Various local and regional flaps for plantar foot reconstruction have been described as well for more extensive wounds. A study by Struckmann and colleagues indicated that both free and pedicled flaps are equally suitable for reconstruction of plantar defects, comparing 12 free flaps with 9 pedicled flaps with no significant difference among functional and long-term results.[32] As the focus of this article is on local pedicled and perforator flaps, following is a description of some of the major local flaps derived from the plantar aspect of the foot.

One viable option for reconstruction of the sole of the foot is a local perforator flap based on the medial plantar artery, also known as the instep flap; this is considered a workhorse option that provides glabrous tissue from the non–weight-bearing medial plantar region for resurfacing of adjacent defects.[33] The flap is based on superficial perforators arising from the superficial branch of the medial plantar artery. This perforator is constant and can be found between the adductor hallucis muscle and the flexor digitorum brevis muscle in proximity to the navicular bone.[33] A cutaneous nerve, a branch of the medial plantar nerve, can provide sensation if incorporated with the flap and can serve as a major advantage.

The reverse sural flap is a well-studied option for reconstruction of lower one-third wounds of the leg, foot, and ankle. The flap is indicated when there is exposed bone without periosteum, hardware, vessels, and tendons in the ankle and heel regions.[34] In regard to the foot, some limitations exist specifically related to its reach; however, the flap can be used to cover medial and lateral malleolar and calcaneal wounds. One advantage of the flap is to provide a well-cushioned weight-bearing surface for calcaneal reconstruction.

The reverse sural flap is based on the sural angiosome and is an interpolated fasciocutaneous flap. The word "reverse" refers to the retrograde blood supply to the flap from the following: perforators from the peroneal and posterior tibial arteries, lesser saphenous vein, and neurocutaneous perforators from the sural nerve. The peroneal artery has 3 to 6 perforators located 4 to 7 cm proximal to the lateral malleolus. The posterior tibial artery has 4 to 5 perforators located 4 to 10 cm above the tip of the medial malleolus.[34] The neurocutaneous perforators around the sural nerve and venocutaneous perforators around the lesser saphenous vein described by Nakajima and colleagues are 2 additional sources for blood supply to the distally based flap that may be included.[34,35] Imanishi and colleagues have demonstrated the lesser saphenous vein, and its collateral veins are the primary venous drainage pathways of the flap.[34,36] As the lesser saphenous vein contains valves, blood flow in a retrograde fashion is believed to be through the smaller collateral veins.

Intrinsic muscle flaps are also powerful for reconstruction. The flexor digitorum brevis flap is a muscular flap option for coverage of small bone exposure.[37] The flap is localized under the plantar aponeurosis, and a sensitive flap can be harvested as well. Circulation to the flap is based off of the lateral plantar artery and can be rotated for assistance with coverage of calcaneal and medial malleolar defects.[37]

The abductor hallucis brevis muscle is a viable and versatile option for reconstruction of various foot and heel defects. It is a muscular flap that arises along the medial border of the foot and has a pedicle derived from branches off the medial plantar artery. The literature describes cases in which the muscle was transposed in combination with a medial plantar artery flap in addition to being used as a distally based turnover flap.[38]

Another alternative for foot reconstruction is the flexor hallucis brevis muscle. This muscular flap has been described as being harvested by itself or in combination with the abductor hallucis brevis from the medial forefoot margin.[39] With the medial plantar artery and first web space artery as its pedicle, its ability to be rotated around the distal forefoot sole on the medial side gives it the potential to aid in coverage of a variety of traumatic and ulcer defects.

RECONSTRUCTION OF THE DORSAL FOOT

Similar to the authors' previous discussion, skin grafting and dermal substitutes should be considered when appropriate for dorsal foot reconstruction. As the goal for dorsal foot reconstruction is to provide a thin, pliable, yet sheer resistant coverage, thinner coverage options should be considered.

When considering local flap coverage, the dorsalis pedis artery flap is a viable option.[40] Sensate and local, this flap is versatile for dorsal foot and ankle coverage. The anterior tibial artery terminates in the dorsalis pedis artery, which divides into the deep plantar artery and the first dorsal metatarsal artery. The dorsal pedis artery also has several cutaneous branches between the extensor retinaculum and the deep plantar branch.[34] With this considered, the dorsal pedis flap represents a viable sensitive fasciocutaneous or myocutaneous flap (including the extensor digitorum brevis muscle) that can be harvested from the dorsum of the foot. Reconstruction of small defects in the distal portion of the foot is a difficult task, but reports of distally based dorsalis pedis fasciocutaneous flaps have been presented in the literature.[41] As a flap that is very thin and supple, which typically fits in its recipient site without bulk, it has also been used extensively for more proximal defects of the ankle and distal portion of the lower leg.

Another option that exists is a flap that can be raised from the dorsum of the foot based distally on the first webspace. It is a fasciocutaneous, sensitive flap with very small dimensions that is supplied by branches of the dorsal and plantar metatarsal arteries and their distal communicating branches. It is a reliable option that is used primarily in resurfacing defects in the distal foot overlying the metatarsophalangeal joints.[42]

RECONSTRUCTION OF THE MEDIAL SIDE OF THE FOOT

Soft tissue defects of the medial side of the foot are difficult to cover adequately, although viable local tissue options do exist for this type of reconstruction. One such example is the medialis pedis flap, which can be based distally on the medial plantar artery of the hallux or the first plantar metatarsal artery perforator.[43] This fasciocutaneous flap can be rotated around the medial malleolar area as well as the Achilles tendon and can also provide coverage for defects of these anatomic locations as well as the posterior aspect of the heel.[44]

RECONSTRUCTION OF THE LATERAL SIDE OF THE FOOT

Posterior heel and lateral foot defects are often difficult to reconstruct, given their osseous bed, poor vascularization, and high functional demands and movement. Conservative treatment often fails, and free flap reconstruction presents a unique challenge. The lateral calcaneal flap based off of the lateral calcaneal artery (terminal branch of peroneal artery) serves as an important surgical option for hindfoot defects. The lateral calcaneal artery is part of a neurovascular bundle that includes the lesser saphenous vein and sural nerve, providing the potential for it to serve as a cutaneous sensitive flap.

Along the lateral aspect of the foot, the abductor digiti minimi muscle serves as a reconstruction for defects along this region of the foot or the lateral malleolar zone. This location is a prominent anatomic structure vulnerable to repetitive trauma and ulcer formation, and the abductor digiti minimi muscle represents a promising treatment option for small- to moderate-sized defects that have exposed bone, joint, or tendon.[37] This muscle flap is larger than the abductor hallucis brevis and receives vascular supply from branches off of the lateral plantar artery.

SUMMARY AND CLINICAL PEARLS

- Lower extremity reconstruction is a continuously evolving field that plays an important part in orthopedic trauma.
- Successful limb salvage requires a coordinated effort of both plastic and orthopedic surgical teams.
- Early consultation to the plastic and reconstructive team will help assist in surgical planning and optimize patient decision-making.
- Reconstruction requires expert knowledge of blood supply to the skin, muscle, and surrounding tissue for success and optimization of soft tissue coverage.
- The thigh is robust in musculature and typically amendable to simple local muscle flap options or just skin grafting.
- The lower leg is divided into thirds (upper, middle, lower) when describing wounds and considering local reconstructive flap options.
- The foot has 7 subunits, and well-reconstructed foot must be able to both tolerate sheering stress force while weight-bearing and adequately contour to accommodate wearing a shoe.
- As techniques and flap utilization continue to improve, the possibilities of soft tissue coverage will evolve and continue to change the landscape of patient-centered conversations regarding limb salvage.

REFERENCES

1. Soltanian H, Garcia RM, Hollenbeck ST. Current Concepts in Lower Extremity Reconstruction. Plast Reconstr Surg 2015;136(6):815e–29e.
2. Lachica RD. Evidence-Based Medicine: Management of Acute Lower Extremity Trauma. Plast Reconstr Surg 2017;139(1):287e–301e.
3. Bosse MJ, MacKenzie EJ, Kellam JF, et al. An analysis of outcomes of reconstruction or amputation after leg-threatening injuries. N Engl J Med 2002;347(24):1924–31.
4. Mendenhall SD, Ben-Amotz O, Gandhi RA, et al. A Review on the Orthoplastic Approach to Lower Limb Reconstruction. Indian J Plast Surg 2019;52(1):17–25.
5. Naga HI, Azoury SC, Othman S, et al. Short- and Long-Term Outcomes following Severe Traumatic Lower Extremity Reconstruction: The Value of an Orthoplastic Limb Salvage Center to Racially Underserved Communities. Plast Reconstr Surg 2021;148(3):646–54.
6. Gustilo RB, Anderson JT. Prevention of infection in the treatment of one thousand and twenty-five open fractures of long bones: retrospective and prospective analyses. J Bone Joint Surg Am 1976;58(4):453–8.
7. Medina ND, Kovach SJ 3rd, Levin LS. An evidence-based approach to lower extremity acute trauma. Plast Reconstr Surg 2011;127(2):926–31.
8. Heller L, Levin LS. Lower extremity microsurgical reconstruction. Plast Reconstr Surg 2001;108(4):1029–41 [quiz: 1042].
9. Reddy V, Stevenson TR. MOC-PS(SM) CME article: lower extremity reconstruction. Plast Reconstr Surg 2008;121(4 Suppl):1–7.
10. MacKenzie EJ, Bosse MJ, Pollak AN, et al. Long-term persistence of disability following severe lower-limb trauma. Results of a seven-year follow-up. J Bone Joint Surg Am 2005;87(8):1801–9.
11. Doukas WC, Hayda RA, Frisch HM, et al. The Military Extremity Trauma Amputation/Limb Salvage (METALS) study: outcomes of amputation versus limb salvage following major lower-extremity trauma. J Bone Joint Surg Am 2013;95(2):138–45.
12. Bosse MJ, Teague D, Reider L, et al. Outcomes After Severe Distal Tibia, Ankle, and/or Foot Trauma: Comparison of Limb Salvage Versus Transtibial Amputation (OUTLET). J Orthop Trauma 2017;31(Suppl 1):S48–s55.
13. Moncrieff M, Hall P. The foot bone's connected to the knee bone": use of the fillet-of-sole flap to avoid an above knee amputation after severe lower limb compartment syndrome. J Trauma 2006;61(5):1264–6.

14. Chiang YC, Wei FC, Wang JW, et al. Reconstruction of below-knee stump using the salvaged foot fillet flap. Plast Reconstr Surg 1995;96(3):731–8.

15. Valerio I, Schulz SA, West J, et al. Targeted Muscle Reinnervation Combined with a Vascularized Pedicled Regenerative Peripheral Nerve Interface. Plast Reconstr Surg Glob Open 2020;8(3):e2689.

16. Hong JP, Hallock GG. Our Premise for Lower Extremity Reconstruction. J Reconstr Microsurg 2021;37(1):1.

17. McCraw JBAPG. McCraw and Arnold's atlas of muscle and musculocutaneous flaps. Norfolk (VA): Hampton Press Pub. Co; 1988.

18. Godina M. Early microsurgical reconstruction of complex trauma of the extremities. Plast Reconstr Surg 1986;78(3):285–92.

19. Lee ZH, Stranix JT, Rifkin WJ, et al. Timing of Microsurgical Reconstruction in Lower Extremity Trauma: An Update of the Godina Paradigm. Plast Reconstr Surg 2019;144(3):759–67.

20. Stannard JP, Volgas DA, Stewart R, et al. Negative pressure wound therapy after severe open fractures: a prospective randomized study. J Orthop Trauma 2009;23(8):552–7.

21. Hassinger SM, Harding G, Wongworawat MD. High-pressure pulsatile lavage propagates bacteria into soft tissue. Clin Orthop Relat Res 2005;439: 27–31.

22. Parrett BM, Matros E, Pribaz JJ, et al. Lower extremity trauma: trends in the management of soft-tissue reconstruction of open tibia-fibula fractures. Plast Reconstr Surg 2006;117(4):1315–22 [discussion: 1323-1314].

23. Cho EH, Shammas RL, Carney MJ, et al. Muscle versus fasciocutaneous free flaps in lower extremity traumatic reconstruction: a multicenter outcomes analysis. Plast Reconstr Surg 2018;141(1):191–9.

24. Engel H, Lin CH, Wei FC. Role of microsurgery in lower extremity reconstruction. Plast Reconstr Surg 2011;127(Suppl 1):228s–38s.

25. AlMugaren FM, Pak CJ, Suh HP, et al. Best Local Flaps for Lower Extremity Reconstruction. Plast Reconstr Surg Glob Open 2020;8(4):e2774.

26. Hallock GG. Sagittal split tibialis anterior muscle flap. Ann Plast Surg 2002;49(1):39–43.

27. Schaverien M, Saint-Cyr M. Perforators of the lower leg: analysis of perforator locations and clinical application for pedicled perforator flaps. Plast Reconstr Surg 2008;122(1):161–70.

28. Mohan AT, Rammos CK, Akhavan AA, et al. Evolving concepts of keystone perforator island flaps (KPIF): principles of perforator anatomy, design modifications, and extended clinical applications. Plast Reconstr Surg 2016;137(6):1909–20.

29. Janis JEGALTSJ. Essentials of plastic surgery. 2014.

30. Crowe CS, Cho DY, Kneib CJ, et al. Strategies for Reconstruction of the Plantar Surface of the Foot: A Systematic Review of the Literature. Plast Reconstr Surg 2019;143(4):1223–44.

31. Hollenbeck ST, Woo S, Komatsu I, et al. Longitudinal outcomes and application of the subunit principle to 165 foot and ankle free tissue transfers. Plast Reconstr Surg 2010;125(3):924–34.

32. Struckmann V, Hirche C, Struckmann F, et al. Free and pedicled flaps for reconstruction of the weight-bearing sole of the foot: a comparative analysis of functional results. J Foot Ankle Surg 2014;53(6): 727–34.

33. Scaglioni MF, Rittirsch D, Giovanoli P. Reconstruction of the heel, middle foot sole, and plantar forefoot with the medial plantar artery perforator flap: clinical experience with 28 cases. Plast Reconstr Surg 2018;141(1):200–8.

34. Follmar KE, Baccarani A, Baumeister SP, et al. The distally based sural flap. Plast Reconstr Surg 2007; 119(6):138e–48e.

35. Nakajima H, Imanishi N, Fukuzumi S, et al. Accompanying arteries of the lesser saphenous vein and sural nerve: anatomic study and its clinical applications. Plast Reconstr Surg 1999;103(1):104–20.

36. Imanishi N, Nakajima H, Fukuzumi S, et al. Venous drainage of the distally based lesser saphenous-sural veno-neuroadipofascial pedicled fasciocutaneous flap: a radiographic perfusion study. Plast Reconstr Surg 1999;103(2):494–8.

37. Hartrampf CR Jr, Scheflan M, Bostwick J 3rd. The flexor digitorum brevis muscle island pedicle flap: a new dimension in heel reconstruction. Plast Reconstr Surg 1980;66(2):264–70.

38. Schwabegger AH, Shafighi M, Gurunluoglu R. Versatility of the abductor hallucis muscle as a conjoined or distally-based flap. J Trauma 2005; 59(4):1007–11.

39. Mahan KT, Feehery RV. Flexor hallucis brevis muscle flap. J Foot Surg 1991;30(3):284–8.

40. Emsen IM. Reconstruction with distally based dorsalis pedis fasciocutaneous flap for the coverage of distal toe-plantar defects. Can J Plast Surg 2012;20(2):e25–27.

41. Krag C, Riegels-Nielsen P. The dorsalis pedis flap for lower leg reconstruction. Acta Orthop Scand 1982;53(3):487–93.

42. Earley MJ, Milner RH. A distally based first web flap in the foot. Br J Plast Surg 1989;42(5):507–11.

43. Park JS, Lee JH, Lee JS, et al. Medialis pedis flap for reconstruction of weight bearing heel. Microsurgery 2017;37(7):780–5.

44. Song D, Yang X, Wu Z, et al. Anatomic basis and clinical application of the distally based medialis pedis flaps. Surg Radiol Anat 2016;38(2):213–21.

Posttraumatic Soft Tissue Coverage of the Lower Leg for the Orthopedic Surgeon

James A. Blair, MD[a],*, George A. Puneky, MD[a],
Thomas E. Dickerson, BS[b], Hayden D. Faith, BS[b],
Jana M. Davis, MD[a]

KEYWORDS

- Rotational flap • Gastrocnemius flap • Soleus flap • Sural flap • Limb salvage

KEY POINTS

- Proximal third lower leg wounds can be reliably covered with a rotational gastrocnemius flap.
- Mid third lower leg wounds can be reliably covered with a rotational soleus flap.
- Distal third lower leg wounds can be reliably covered with a reverse sural fasciocutaneous flap provided the most distal lateral perforator is still intact..
- Soft tissue coverage of lower extremity wounds with rotational flaps can be performed by an orthopaedic surgeon without need for loupes or a microscope.

INTRODUCTION

Lower extremity fractures are common to the practicing orthopedic surgeon. It has been estimated that soft tissue injuries are present in up to 82.8% of traumatized orthopedic patients.[1] Although there is a broad spectrum of soft tissue injury, some may require advanced coverage techniques beyond primary wound closure.[2] Failure to adequately address soft tissue injury may result in poor outcomes, such as the development of infection, complicating limb salvage, and increasing risk of future amputation. Advances in the understanding of vascular anatomy and the development of wound adjuncts, such as negative pressure wound therapy (NPWT), have allowed surgeons to enhance their treatment efficacy for a variety of lower extremity wounds.[3–5]

Time to coverage is critical, with recent studies demonstrating soft tissue coverage within 3 days of injury, and/or immediately following fracture fixation, substantially decreases wound infection rates.[6] The ability of the orthopedic surgeon to be well versed in different forms of wound management negates the reliance on interdisciplinary teams and subsequent delays in definitive coverage that may ensue. A recent international survey of 51 orthopedic surgeons estimated that more than 93% of 970 amputations performed over a 1-year span were the result of inadequate education in soft tissue injury management.[7] Soft tissue coverage procedures are not technically difficult or resource demanding and can significantly reduce disability-adjusted life years when performed early.[7]

Soft tissue reconstruction aims to close wounds, promote revascularization of ischemic tissue, prevent infection, limit nonunion, and ultimately prevent amputation.[8] Adjuncts, like NPWT, have allowed more leniency with wound coverage delays following fracture fixation without altering patient outcome.[9] Techniques such as piecrusting have improved the ability to primarily close wounds despite significant edema, reducing the need for skin grafts.[10] The application of split thickness skin grafts

[a] Department of Orthopedic Surgery, Medical College of Georgia at Augusta University, 1120 15th St., BA 3300, Augusta, GA 30912, USA; [b] Medical College of Georgia at Augusta University, 1120 15th Street, Augusta, GA 30912, USA
* Corresponding author.
E-mail address: jamblair@augusta.edu
Twitter: @jamesablairMD (J.A.B.); @janadavisMD (J.M.D.)

Orthop Clin N Am 53 (2022) 297–310
https://doi.org/10.1016/j.ocl.2022.03.002
0030-5898/22/

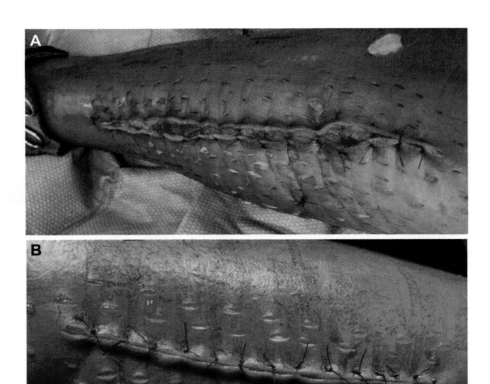

Fig. 1. (*A, B*) Piecrusting technique demonstrating successful primary closure of a medial leg fasciotomy skin incision in 2 different patients. Any gaps in closure were allowed to heal by secondary intention. No skin grafts were required. (*Courtesy of* Frank R. Arko, MD.)

(STSG) has allowed for superficial wound coverage in the presence of skin defects. Techniques in rotational flap coverage have been revolutionary in the management of traumatic wounds to the lower extremity. Gastrocnemius flaps offer a reliable and versatile option for coverage over the knee and proximal third of the lower extremity without requiring highly specialized microsurgical intervention.[11] Soleus and hemisoleus flaps have simplified coverage of defects overlying the anterior middle third of the lower leg. Reverse sural artery flaps (RSAF) allow coverage of the distal third of the lower leg, ankle, and foot.[12] The following sections describe these procedures and highlight the importance of the orthopedic surgeon to acquire and perform these skills.

Adjuncts to Assist Wound Closure

Wounds may be primarily closed in a delayed manner to survey for the onset of infection and/or progressive tissue necrosis as a traumatic wound evolves. Delayed primary wound closure

(DPWC) may be implemented after adequate debridement in contaminated wounds or when initial swelling/edema restricts proper wound closure.[13] Although this technique can prove beneficial, comorbidities affecting proper wound closure should be taken into consideration (ie, diabetes, renal failure, smoking).[14]

NPWT, also known as vacuum-assisted closure or microdeformational wound therapy, has transformed the landscape of wound care over the past 25 years.[15] An NPWT dressing consists of a sterile sponge that is placed into the wound bed and covered with an impermeable film. A suction tube is windowed into the impermeable film to allow drainage into an external fluid canister.[15] This technique uses subatomospheric pressure to introduce microdeformation and increase the formation of granulation tissue, eliminating dead space, and facilitating wound healing or closure. NPWT was first described in 1997 as a means to treat "chronic and difficult-to-manage wounds."[16] Since introduction, NPWT has become a widely accepted practice in wound treatment. In a meta-analysis comparing NPWT to conventional wound dressing for open fractures, NPWT showed reduced infection rate, shorter healing time and length of hospital stay, and lower rate of amputation.[17,18] However, another study investigating disability following treatment of severe open fracture of the lower limb with NPWT compared with standard wound therapy demonstrated no statistical difference in patient-reported disability outcomes at 12 months.[19]

Some traumatic wounds or surgical incisions may not be amenable to DPWC. The technique of piecrusting may be performed when skin edges are unable to be reapproximated without undue tension due to skin loss or edema. Piecrusting facilitates primary closure by relieving superficial skin tension via creation of multiple subcentimeter incisions parallel to a wound or incision (**Fig. 1**). Rows of piecrusting perforations are generally performed along both sides of a tensioned skin incision, with the first row placed 10 to 20 mm from the skin edge. Each perforation is approximately 10 to 15 mm in length and must be through the dermis while being at least 10 mm apart. Subsequent piecrusting rows are added as necessary relative to the amount of tension and are typically staggered from the previous row. A single row has been shown to decrease wound tension by an average of 34%.[10] Decreasing skin tension in high-risk areas of the leg (ie, adjacent to the ankle) can reduce the rate of wound dehiscence, infection,[20] and the need for STSG.[10] Studies have shown that this technique may be implemented with minimal scarring or patient morbidity.[10,20]

Split Thickness Skin Grafts

Primary closure may not be an option with increasing wound size and complexity. Wounds with underlying vascularized tissue may be managed in the form of superficial skin coverage using STSG. An STSG is composed of both the epidermis and a small portion of the underlying dermis. Retention of most of the dermis at the donor site improves healing by allowing reepithelization to occur, decreasing autograft morbidity. STSG can be taken from a multitude of locations, with lateral thigh and trunk being the most common autograft sites.[21] Graft thickness can be classified as thin (0.15–0.3 mm), intermediate (0.3–0.45 mm), or thick (0.45–0.6 mm).[22] STSG success relies on the vascularity of the wound bed. Thicker grafts, although more robust, require more extensive vascularity for successful wound healing.[21] Contraindications include inadequate wound bed vascularization, exposed tendon or bone, active infection, a

wound overlying a joint, or an actively bleeding wound.[21] Common comorbidities such as tobacco use, chronic steroid use, and diabetes can prevent successful grafting but are not in themselves considered contraindications.

Technique

Following wound debridement and irrigation, the site is evaluated for appropriateness to receive skin graft and ensure a suitable soft tissue bed. Wound margins without significant tension are closed primarily with the intention of decreasing the size of the required graft. The defect size is measured using a sterile ruler and the skin graft donor site is templated, most commonly along the anterolateral thigh. The donor site is prepared using mineral oil to reduce dermatome friction. The dermatome is set to a graft depth of 0.015 to 0.018 in, which may be confirmed as the depth required to accommodate a #10 scalpel. The dermatome is positioned at a less than 45° angle at the leading edge of the donor site and translated, using steady pressure, to the desired graft dimensions. The end edge of the graft is truncated using a scalpel. The graft may be processed through a mesher to increase graft area and pliability. In addition, meshing allows fluid egress through the graft, thereby preventing hematoma formation, which may lead to graft failure. Meshing to a larger scale may accommodate a larger wound coverage per graft size, but can result in contracture during epithelialization. The graft is sutured or stapled in place over the wound bed (dermal side down). A nonstick dressing (ie, Adaptic or Xeroform) is placed over the STSG. Alternatively, an NPWT dressing may be used over the graft site to reduce graft shear, improve graft adherence, and decrease hematoma formation. The initial dressing may be left in place for up to 7 days before transitioning to dry dressings. A single-ply Xeroform gauze dressing is placed over the donor site and is maintained in place until healing has occurred.

Clinics Care Points

- Mineral oil should be used to reduce friction during graft harvest.

- Meshing graft to a 1:1.5 scale increases size and pliability

- Graft should be placed dermal side down over wound bed.

- Donor site dressing should remain in place until healing has occurred.

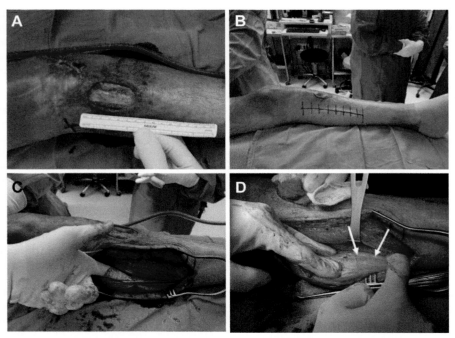

Fig. 2. (A–D) Medial gastrocnemius flap of a single patient. (A) Measurement of pretibial defect following debridement. (B) An incision is marked out along the posteromedial border of the tibia. (C) Plantaris tendon localized to identify correct plane between gastrocnemius and soleus. (D) Identification of the raphe (arrow) separating the medial and lateral heads of the gastrocnemius.

LOWER LEG ROTATIONAL FLAPS

Complex soft tissue defects of the lower extremity with exposed tendon, bone, or implants create unique situations in which simple means of soft tissue coverage (ie, DPWC or STSG) will result in clinical failure. Musculofasciocutaneous flaps are preferred in these situations and provide advantages including improved rates of functional healing, resistance to trauma, and cosmetic appearance.[11] The use of local muscle flaps was first described in 1946,[23] and advancement with these techniques have shown favor, relative to free flaps, because local rotational flaps negate the need for microsurgery, specialized equipment, and long operating times.[11] The ability to perform rotational flaps without the need for microvascular surgical techniques is a powerful tool for the orthopedic surgeon treating such injuries. Common contraindications to coverage by rotational flap include active infection, flap reach limitations, compromised extremity perfusion, and patient factors contributing to an inability to safely undergo surgery or heal the surgical site.[24,25] Different rotational flap techniques have been described and applied in clinical practice to provide soft tissue coverage from the knee to the heel. Here the authors further describe the application of the gastrocnemius and soleus rotational muscle flaps, and the reverse sural artery rotational fasciocutaneous flap.

Rotational Gastrocnemius Flaps

Gastrocnemius flaps offer a versatile option for coverage over both the knee and proximal third of the lower leg. First described in 1978, this technique was later applied in 1981 to provide coverage over a knee prosthesis, and in 1984 for posttumor reconstruction.[26–28] The medial and lateral heads of the gastrocnemius muscle receive arterial flow from the medial and lateral sural arteries, respectively. The proximal location of the arterial pedicle allows for distal detachment and rotation of the muscle from the triceps surae, reaching up to 15 cm from the knee joint.[24]

General indications for gastrocnemius flaps include soft tissue defects around the knee or proximal third tibia with exposed bone, tendon, joint capsule, cartilage, or implants.[24] In situations in which a slight increase in flap width is desired, fenestration or excision of the superficial and/or deep fascia may be performed. When greater excursion is required, further detachment of the origin of the gastrocnemius from the distal femur may be performed, provided the arterial blood supply is not jeopardized. Larger defects overlying fracture may be amenable to rotational gastrocnemius flaps after creation of an intentional shortening and angular deformity, with intent to later perform gradual deformity correction in a circular frame.[23] Medial gastrocnemius flaps are often used in practice given their larger size and excursion. The lateral gastrocnemius flap is limited in size and mobility due to the common peroneal nerve crossing over the pedicle and the need to travel over the proximal fibula.[29]

Technique

The patient is positioned supine and draped to expose the entire lower extremity to the hip (Fig. 2). A tourniquet is typically not required. A straight medial incision is started at the knee joint line and continued distally for 12 to 15 cm along the posterior border of the tibia. The saphenous vein is identified, and small branches are cauterized to allow mobilization. The subcutaneous tissue is dissected until the gastrocnemius fascia is identified. The gastrocnemius fascia is incised at its most medial point. The triceps surae tendon is identified distally. The gastrocnemius is mobilized with blunt dissection between the gastrocnemius muscle belly, overlying subcutaneous tissue, and soleus. The plantaris tendon is identified between the gastrocnemius and soleus and serves as a marker to ensure the correct interval. Blunt dissection is continued laterally until identification of the gastrocnemius raphe between the medial and lateral heads. Commonly, this cannot be delineated on the undersurface (deep aspect) of the muscle fascia but can be identified from the superficial aspect. Curved Mayo scissors are used to transect the distal gastrocnemius tendon, proximal to its insertion into the triceps surae tendon, and curved proximally to the central raphe. It is important to not complete the gastrocnemius tenotomy in a transverse fashion because this will detach the lateral head from the remainder of the triceps surae tendon. The dissection is carried proximally following the raphe. Once the bulk of the muscle belly is encountered, the dissection can usually be completed bluntly. A critical maneuver is to continue this dissection to the origin of the gastrocnemius at the level of the distal femur; this ensures supple excursion of the muscle and allows coverage of more proximal and lateral wounds. When done carefully, the vasculature of the medial head is readily preserved.

The medial head of the gastrocnemius is now free to rotate to the desired position. If more surface area is required, the deep and superficial fascia can be fenestrated to allow the muscle belly to flatten. Manual manipulation is best, and forceps/pickups should be avoided because instruments may unintentionally crush the muscle tissue resulting in local necrosis. When treating more central or lateral wounds, the decision to tunnel the flap under a skin bridge should be made at this point. An elevator is used to create a tunnel above the periosteum or fascia for flap passage under the skin and into the defect. Care must be taken to ensure enough tissue is released so as to not strangulate the flap. If tunneling is not desired, a transverse incision is made along the skin where the muscle flap will lie. Once the flap is rotated, the skin is closed primarily over the inset flap. Healthy skin and subcutaneous tissue should overlie the flap periphery. The wound skin edges are elevated to allow at least 15 mm of flap inlay. Multiple modified Mason-Allen stitches are placed along the periphery of the muscle flap (Fig. 3) using nonabsorbable suture (the authors prefer a 0 Prolene suture because it is a different color than standard nylon suture and easier to identify which sutures must remain in place during postoperative visits). Once the desired position for the muscle flap is determined, a free needle is used to bring the sutures out of the skin, from deep to proximal, and the sutures are tied to each other over the skin. Bolsters may be used to protect the skin. These sutures should remain in place for a minimum of 6 weeks. The overlying skin is secured into place using 3-0 chromic gut suture with subcutaneous or simple interrupted stitches. The initial surgical incision is closed primarily. An STSG is placed over any exposed muscle. Weight-bearing as tolerated from a soft tissue standpoint may be allowed around 3 weeks postoperatively once the incisions have healed. The leg is maintained in neutral elevation with respect to the heart. Anecdotally, postoperative protocols involving extremity heating and intentional lowering of the extremity below the heart have shown to be unnecessary.

Clinics Care Points

- Separate the raphe proximally to the level of the distal femur.
- Fenestration of the superficial and deep fascia allows flattening of the muscle, increasing surface area.
- Grabbing the muscle belly with pickups or forceps may cause local necrosis.

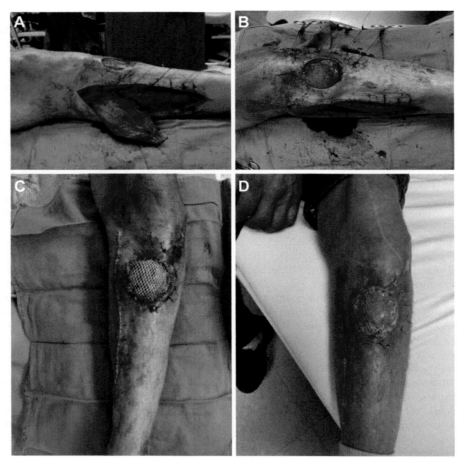

Fig. 3. (A–D) Flap rotation and postoperative images of the same patient as in **Fig. 2.** (A) A distally free medial gastrocnemius flap with modified Mason-Allen stitches placed along the periphery. (B) The flap is tunneled and rotated into position. (C) Closure of medial surgical wound and placement of STSG over the muscle flap. (D) Six-week postoperative photograph displaying successful defect closure.

- Ensure adequate tunneling to prevent flap congestion.
- Inlay the flap to allow healthy skin to overlie the muscle belly.
- Use nonabsorbable suture to secure the flap and remove 6 weeks postoperatively.
- Flap bulk will decrease over time as muscle atrophy occurs.

Soleus/Hemisoleus Flaps

The soleus flap has shown practicality over time as good coverage option over the anterior middle third of the leg, dating back to reports published in 1973.[23] The soleus muscle is a large, bipennate muscle along the posterior aspect of the leg. The medial portion of the soleus is supplied by perforators originating from the posterior tibial artery, making the soleus muscle a reliable option for a proximally or distally based pedicle flap.[26] However, the variable amount of lower soleus perforators from the peroneal artery results in a less predictable distally based pedicle flap.[26] A defined intermuscular septum separates the medial and lateral portions of the soleus muscle, allowing for a hemisoleus flap to be harvested, which can be used for less extensive injuries within reach.[27] In general, common contraindications to flap reconstruction apply to soleus flaps.[28]

Technique

The patient is positioned supine and draped to expose the entire lower extremity to the hip (**Fig. 4**). A hip bump is not placed, preserving exposure to the medial aspect of the leg. A sterile tourniquet may be placed, if desired. A 15-cm incision is made 2 cm posterior to the posteromedial border of the tibia. The superficial

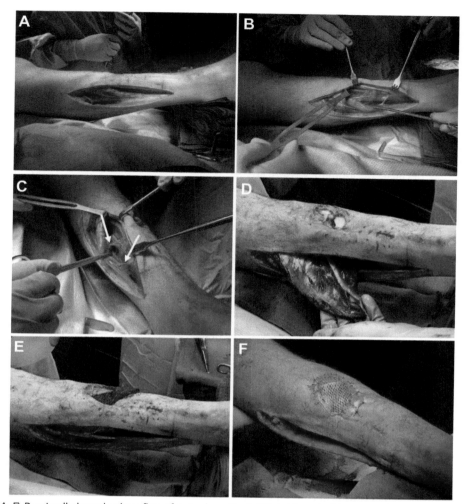

Fig. 4. (*A–F*) Proximally based soleus flap of a single patient: (*A*) A 15-cm incision is made 2 cm posterior to the posteromedial border of the tibia in the center of the leg. (*B*) The gastrocnemius is dissected off the posterior soleus fascia; note the plantaris tendon adherent to the deep surface of the gastrocnemius fascia. (*C*) Perforating arteries are identified and signified by arrows. (*D*) The soleus is transected from the Achilles tendon distally. (*E*) The flap is tunneled to the wound bed subcutaneously. (*F*) STSG is used for coverage over muscle flap. (*Courtesy of* Joseph R. Hsu, MD.)

compartment fascia will be visible following incision of skin and subcutaneous tissue. A longitudinal incision is made through the superficial compartment fascia, in line with the skin incision, to expose the gastrocnemius and soleus muscles more proximally and the triceps surae tendon distally.

The soleus must next be identified on both its superficial and deep surfaces. First, the plane between the soleus and gastrocnemius fascia is identified using sharp dissection. Visualization of the plantaris tendon within this interval helps to ensure the surgeon is in the correct plane. The gastrocnemius is elevated from the soleus the full width of the muscle, both proximally

and distally, until the triceps surae origin is visualized. It is the author's preferred technique to rotate the full soleus rather than a hemisoleus, although a hemisoleus flap may be performed if desired.

Next, the soleus must be elevated from the deep posterior compartment. The deep posterior compartment fascia is readily seen in the distal extent of the incision located anterior and deep to the soleus. Care must be taken not to enter the deep posterior compartment by violating the overlying fascia during dissection. The soleus is then sharply elevated from the deep posterior compartment distally, making sure to identify any perforating vessels from the peroneal artery piercing the fascia and supplying the soleus muscle. To create a proximally based flap, the most distal perforators will be ligated with either vascular clips or 2-0 silk ties before transection. The soleus is then transected in its entirety as distally as possible, making sure the Achilles tendon remains intact. The flap may then be raised from distal to proximal. In the more proximal extent of the leg, the soleus must be elevated from its fibular origin. Flap excursion is continually checked in relation to the wound because perforating vessels are divided to limit the number of perforators sacrificed to obtain flap rotation. One should avoid dissecting more proximally than what is necessary to preserve the more proximal perforating arteries, which supply blood flow to the flap.

The flap is tunneled to the wound bed subcutaneously, ensuring there are no points of flap constriction during rotation. If tunneling results in flap constriction, an incision overlying the area of rotation must be made. Skin flaps can be elevated to allow safe passage of the soleus into the wound bed. Simple, nonabsorbent sutures are circumferentially placed through the skin into the soleus fascia to maintain flap position. An STSG is placed over the muscle and secured in place with staples. NPWT or a bolster dressing is placed over the skin graft for 5 to 7 days before removal. The medial incision is closed primarily.

In cases in which more distal coverage is desired, a distally based rotational flap may be performed. After identifying and isolating the soleus, the soleus remains attached to its distal perforators and is transected proximally. Care must be taken to prevent transection of the perforators in the distal aspect of the flap as they are fewer than the proximal perforators. Similar to the gastrocnemius flap postoperative protocol, the extremity is maintained at neutral elevation with respect to the heart and adjuncts such as extremity heating are not required. Patients may be advanced to weight-bearing as tolerated from a soft tissue standpoint around 3 weeks postoperatively once the incisions have healed.

Clinics Care Points

- Plan to perform soleus versus hemisoleus flap is decided once the soleus muscle is exposed.
- Evaluate proximal and distal perforators before vessel ligation for determination of flap base.
- Minimize number of perforators ligated.

- Be aware of any flap constriction points that may lead to failure.
- Limit handling the muscle tissue with forceps.
- The soleus is typically not as robust as the gastrocnemius.

Reverse Sural Artery Flap

Distal wounds of the lower extremity offer a unique challenge to the orthopedic surgeon due to soft tissue stress secondary to weight-bearing, the subcutaneous nature of bone in this area, and the lack of local muscle tissue.[29] Common teaching is wounds in this area require free tissue transfer; however, the RSAF is a neurofasciocutaneous flap that has demonstrated utility for coverage of the distal third of the lower extremity, the ankle, and the posterior heel.[30] This technique originated in 1981 as a fasciocutaneous flap[31] and evolved over the years as the sural nerve was incorporated into the dissection,[32] followed by the introduction of a rotational component in 2004.[25] The RSAF is not as robust as the gastrocnemius or soleus flaps because it does not include any muscle tissue in the wound bed, although it does provide a means of local soft tissue coverage without the need for microsurgery. The RSAF relies on perforating branches from the peroneal artery and medial sural artery, typically arising laterally, avoiding sacrifice of deeper arterial structures. Recent anatomic dissections have even described a new blood supply from the lateral retromalleolar perforator of the peroneal artery usually located 1 cm above the lateral malleolus.[33]

The RSAF is indicated for defects within 10 cm of the foot or ankle region, although the authors have anecdotally used the RSAF for midtibial soft tissue defects with success. This technique is especially advantageous because it avoids sacrifice of the 3 main arteries of the leg.[12] It is important to consider patient risk factors because diabetes mellitus, peripheral vascular disease, and venous insufficiency have been linked to a 30% complication rate.[12] Flap viability may be improved using techniques such as flap delay,[34] wide pedicle harvest,[35] and supercharging. The supercharging technique involves elevating the proposed flap and cutting the sural neurovascular bundle without harvesting the pedicle.[11] The pedicle is allowed to sit for 5 to 7 days before pedicle harvest and flap mobilization; this increases vascular flow to the flap from the pedicle and may improve flap success when concern for violation

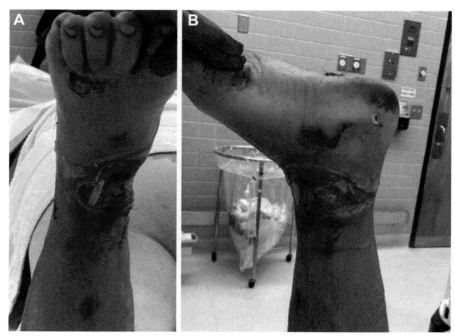

Fig. 5. (*A, B*) A left-sided distal tibial defect with a single patient in the prone position and the knee flexed.

of the lateral perforators exists (ie, lateral leg incision for fibula fracture fixation or a lateral ankle wound).

Technique

The patient is positioned prone or in lateral decubitus position depending on the location of the soft tissue defect (Fig. 5). A transverse line is drawn along the posterior skin 5 cm proximal to the tip of the lateral malleolus to create a "no-fly zone" (NFZ) in which no subfascial dissection should be performed distal to this mark to protect the last reliable lateral perforating artery. The soft tissue defect is sharply rounded off with a scalpel to allow for easier creation of the flap shape, and the required dimensions are measured. The authors prefer to trace the shape of the defect using the paper that comes standard with sterile gloves and use this when anticipating pedicle length. A sterile paper ruler is used for planning purposes to mimic the pedicle. One end of the ruler is placed in the center posterior aspect of the leg, and the tracing paper is attached to the other end. Multiple pedicle lengths are trialed until an appropriate length is found that minimizes tension. If the pedicle is to make a 180° turn, an extra 1 cm of length is added to the pedicle. Once the appropriate pedicle length is determined, the proposed flap donor site is traced out with a marking pen on the posterior calf (Fig. 6).

Two longitudinal lines are drawn on the skin to mark out a 4-cm pedicle width from the NFZ line to the inferior aspect of the proposed flap. A third line directly between these lines should be drawn from the NFZ to the inferior aspect of the flap. A superficial incision is made along the flap borders as well as the central longitudinal line. A subdermal dissection, distal to the flap paddle, is carried out symmetrically to the edges of the 4-cm pedicle width lines. This is typically performed with a #15 blade with "feathering" strokes to the subdermal tissue. A transverse superficial incision can be made along the NFZ line to aid in subdermal flaps. A similar transverse incision can be made at the inferior margin of the flap to complete the subdermal flaps (Fig. 7).

A standard skin incision is made along the remainder of the flap starting at the edge of the 4-cm pedicle width line and progressing along the upper three-quarters of the flap. The sural neurovascular bundle will be encountered at the proximal apex of this incision. A traction neurectomy of the sural nerve can be performed, and the vasculature is ligated or cauterized. A fascial incision is made along the flap outline. The adventitial tissue deep to the fascial layer of the flap is used as a blunt dissection plane. The decision to supercharge the flap must be made at this point before pedicle harvesting (Fig. 8). If supercharging is desired, the

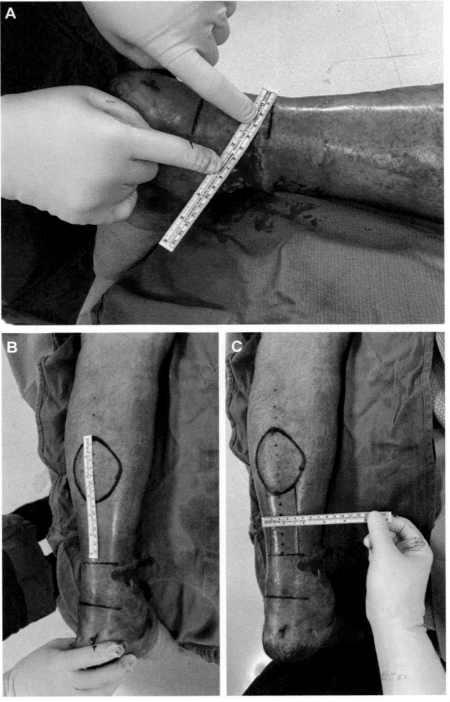

Fig. 6. (A–C) Reverse sural artery flap preparation for the same patient as in Fig. 5. (A) A sterile paper ruler is used to mimic the pedicle and estimate the required length. (B) Templated pedicle dimensions with demarcation of the NFZ 5 cm proximal to the tip of the lateral malleolus. (C) Two longitudinal lines are drawn on the skin to mark out a 4 cm pedicle width.

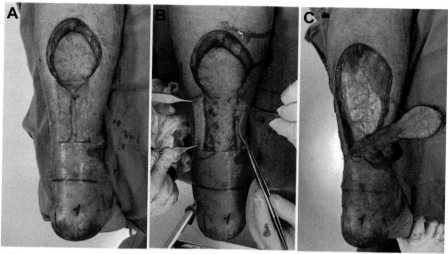

Fig. 7. (*A–C*) Intraoperative photographs of the same patient as in **Fig. 5** and **6.** (*A*) A superficial incision is made along the flap borders as well as the central longitudinal line. (*B*) Subdermal dissection is carried out to the edges of the 4-cm pedicle width lines to create symmetric subdermal flaps. (*C*) A fascial incision is carried along the limits of the subdermal dissection, maintaining the pedicle width. The adventitial layer of the subfascial tissue is bluntly dissected and lifted off the posterior aspect of the Achilles tendon.

dissection is halted and the skin is tacked closed with suture for a 5- to 7-day latency period before flap harvest and wound coverage. Skin necrosis would be noted following the latency period in the event the flap did not survive being cut off from the sural vascular bundle. If supercharging failure has occurred, the iatrogenic wound is debrided and covered using STSG. Additionally, an RSAF is not possible in this situation and other means of coverage must be considered. A flap that survives division from its sural vasculature is enhanced by increased pedicle blood flow. Once the flap is elevated to the leading edge of the subdermal dissection in the distal one-quarter of the flap paddle, the fascial incision is carried distally, medially, and laterally. While maintaining a 4 cm width at all times, the adventitial layer of the subfascial tissue can be blunted dissected and lifted off the posterior aspect of the Achilles tendon. Dissection is continued distally to the level of the NFZ, thus creating the pedicle.

The flap can be rotated to fit over the soft tissue defect (**Fig. 9**). If tunneling is desired, the subcutaneous tunnel must be wide enough to allow easy passage of the flap paddle and avoid vascular constriction. If tunneling is not desired or not possible, a transverse incision is made through the subcutaneous tissue overlaid by the pedicle. This soft tissue can be brought back over the pedicle and loosely approximated, if desired. The flap is secured into place with a combination of 3-0 nylon and 3-0 chromic gut sutures

in a simple interrupted or subcutaneous manner. Caution must be exercised not to place the skin under undue tension in the setting of a flap/donor thickness mismatch. It is better to leave exposed subcutaneous tissue than risk flap edge necrosis.

The pedicle donor site is primarily closed and the flap donor site may sometimes be reapproximated. If not, an STSG may be placed over the adventitial tissue overlying the Achilles tendon or gastrocnemius muscle belly. Any exposed tissue of the pedicle should be covered with an STSG. The ankle is typically immobilized in a splint for soft tissue rest and to minimize shear across the flap and skin graft sites.

CLINICS CARE POINTS

- Maintain pedicle width of 4 cm to minimize flap failure and recheck during harvest.
- Exercise caution not to peel the flap away from its underlying fascia. The fascia must stay with the flap.
- Once the fascial incisions are made for the flap, minimize handling of the flap paddle.
- Avoid tension at the flap skin edges, otherwise edge necrosis may occur.
- Avoid vascular congestion if tunneling the flap/pedicle.

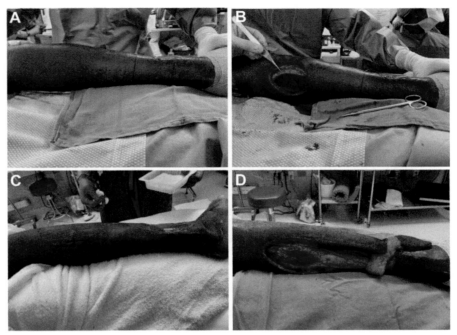

Fig. 8. (A–D) RSAF supercharge in the presence of a lateral ankle wound. The patient is positioned in the lateral decubitus. (A) The skin is marked for the proposed flap. (B) Only the flap paddle is incised through the fascia. The sural neurovascular bundle is transected. (C) The skin is reapproximated and the flap allowed to sit for 5 days. (D) The pedicle is harvested and the flap rotated on a return trip to the operating room.

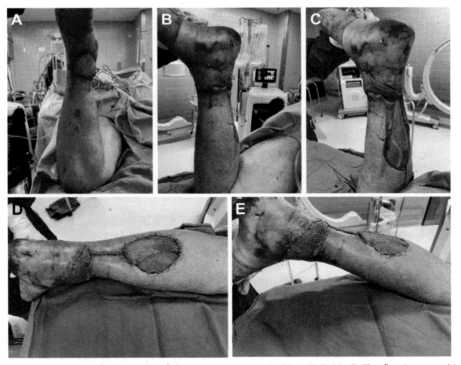

Fig. 9. (A–E) Intraoperative photographs of the same patient as in Figs. 5–7. (A–C) The flap is rotated into place and secured with suture. (D, E) STSG is placed over exposed muscle and pedicle.

SUMMARY

Lower extremity trauma care is common with many patients presenting with complex soft tissue injuries. Many orthopedic surgeons perceive such soft tissue injuries to be out of their scope of practice due to presumed complexity and need for microsurgical and vascular reconstructive techniques. In this review, common approaches to treating these injuries and the ease with which these skills may be acquired and executed are discussed. Neither microsurgery nor vascular surgery is required. Methods such as DPWC, NPWT, and piecrusting serve to decrease wound tension and increase rates of successful healing through primary closure. Superficial wound coverage with STSG can provide appropriate coverage in situations in which primary wound closure is unable be obtained. As wound complexity increases, local rotational soft tissue flaps may be necessary to cover exposed bone, tendon, or implants. A multitude of courses are available in the United States and abroad to provide education in wound coverage such as The Surgical Management and Reconstructive Training (SMART) Course, Advanced Techniques in the Management of Soft Tissue (AO North America), and the Soft Tissue Coverage Skills Course (Orthopaedic Trauma Association and Limb Lengthening and Reconstruction Society). The gastrocnemius, soleus, and reverse sural artery rotational flaps prove highly resourceful to the orthopedic surgeon and negate the need for microsurgery or potential delays when working with a multidisciplinary team.

DISCLOSURE

Dr J.A. Blair is a consultant for Stryker, Inc; Smith & Nephew, Inc; Integra Lifesciences Corporation; and NuVasive Specialized Orthopedics. The remaining authors have no relevant financial disclosures.

CLINICS CARE POINTS

- Soft tissue injury is prevalent in lower extremity trauma
- Management of soft tissues adjacent to fracture can dictate patient outcomes
- Orthopedic surgeons can be equipped to care for soft tissue defects
- Coverage of many lower extremity soft tissue wounds does not necessitate vascular or microvascular techniques

- A variety of skin closure methods and rotational flaps are useful tools to the orthopedic surgeon

REFERENCES

1. Albright PD, Mackechnie MC, Jackson JH, et al. Knowledge deficits and barriers to performing soft-tissue coverage procedures: An analysis of participants in an orthopaedic surgical skills training course in Mexico. OTA Int 2019;2(4):e044.
2. Cierny G 3rd, Byrd HS, Jones RE. Primary versus delayed soft tissue coverage for severe open tibial fractures. a comparison of results. Clin Orthop Relat Res 1983;178:54–63.
3. Liu DS, Sofiadellis F, Ashton M, MacGill K, Webb A. Early soft tissue coverage and negative pressure wound therapy optimises patient outcomes in lower limb trauma. Injury 2012;43(6):772–8.
4. Janis JE, Kwon RK, Attinger CE. The new reconstructive ladder: modifications to the traditional model. Plast Reconstr Surg 2011;127(Suppl 1):205s–12s.
5. Bhattacharyya T, Mehta P, Smith M, Pomahac B. Routine use of wound vacuum-assisted closure does not allow coverage delay for open tibia fractures. Plast Reconstr Surg 2008;121(4):1263–6.
6. Godina M. Early microsurgical reconstruction of complex trauma of the extremities. Plast Reconstr Surg 1986;78(3):285–92.
7. Wu HH, Patel KR, Caldwell AM, Coughlin RR, Hansen SL, Carey JN. Surgical management and reconstruction training (SMART) course for international orthopedic surgeons. Ann Glob Health 2016; 82(4):652–8.
8. Pollak AN, McCarthy ML, Burgess AR. Short-term wound complications after application of flaps for coverage of traumatic soft-tissue defects about the tibia. the lower extremity assessment project (LEAP) study group. J Bone Joint Surg Am 2000; 82(12):1681–91.
9. Zeiderman MR, Pu LLQ. Contemporary approach to soft-tissue reconstruction of the lower extremity after trauma. Burns Trauma 2021;9:tkab024.
10. Capo J, Liporace F, Yingling JM, et al. Pressure reducing skin pie-crusting in extremity trauma: An in-vitro biomechanical study and human case series. Injury 2020;51(6):1266–70.
11. Tan O, Atik B, Bekerecioglu M. Supercharged reverse-flow sural flap: a new modification increasing the reliability of the flap. Microsurgery 2005;25(1):36–43.
12. Ciofu RN, Zamfirescu DG, Popescu SA, Lascar I. Reverse sural flap for ankle and heel soft tissues reconstruction. J Med Life 2017;10(1):94–8.
13. Dimick AR. Delayed wound closure: indications and techniques. Ann Emerg Med 1988;17(12):1303–4.

14. Mankowitz SL. Laceration management. J Emerg Med 2017;53(3):369–82.

15. Huang C, Leavitt T, Bayer LR, Orgill DP. Effect of negative pressure wound therapy on wound healing. Curr Probl Surg 2014;51(7):301–31.

16. Argenta LC, Morykwas MJ. Vacuum-assisted closure: a new method for wound control and treatment: clinical experience. Ann Plast Surg 1997; 38(6):563–76. discussion 577.

17. Liu X, Zhang H, Cen S, Huang F. Negative pressure wound therapy versus conventional wound dressings in treatment of open fractures: a systematic review and meta-analysis. Int J Surg 2018;53: 72–9.

18. Pappalardo V, Frattini F, Ardita V, Rausei S. Negative pressure therapy (NPWT) for management of surgical wounds: effects on wound healing and analysis of devices evolution. Surg Technol Int 2019;34:56–67.

19. Costa ML, Achten J, Bruce J, et al. Effect of negative pressure wound therapy vs standard wound management on 12-month disability among adults with severe open fracture of the lower limb: the wollf randomized clinical trial. JAMA 2018;319(22): 2280–8.

20. Singh D, Lomax A. Piecrusting to facilitate skin closure. Foot Ankle Spec 2016;9(4):367–71.

21. Braza ME, Fahrenkopf MP. Split-Thickness Skin Grafts [Updated 2021 Jul 31]. In: StatPeals [Internet]. Treasure Island (FL): StatPearls Publishing; 2022.

22. Taylor BC, Triplet JJ, Wells M. Split-thickness skin grafting: a primer for orthopaedic surgeons. J Am Acad Orthop Surg 2021;29(20):855–61.

23. Fang F, Chung KC. An evolutionary perspective on the history of flap reconstruction in the upper extremity. Hand Clin 2014;30(2):109–22, v.

24. Pers M, Medgyesi S. Pedicle muscle flaps and their applications in the surgery of repair. Br J Plast Surg 1973;26(4):313–21.

25. Chang SM, Zhang F, Yu GR, Hou CL, Gu YD. Modified distally based peroneal artery perforator flap for reconstruction of foot and ankle. Microsurgery 2004;24(6):430–6.

26. Raveendran SS, Kumaragama KG. Arterial supply of the soleus muscle: anatomical study of fifty lower limbs. Clin Anat 2003;16(3):248–52.

27. Song P, Pu LLQ. The soleus muscle flap: an overview of its clinical applications for lower extremity reconstruction. Ann Plast Surg 2018;81(6S Suppl 1):S109–16.

28. Hankiss J, Schmitz C. [The soleus muscle flap]. Oper Orthop Traumatol 2013;25(2):145–51. Die Musculus-soleus-Lappenplastik.

29. Chang SM, Li XH, Gu YD. Distally based perforator sural flaps for foot and ankle reconstruction. World J Orthop 2015;6(3):322–30.

30. Johnson L, Liette MD, Green C, Rodriguez P, Masadeh S. The reverse sural artery flap: a reliable and versatile flap for wound coverage of the distal lower extremity and hindfoot. Clin Podiatr Med Surg 2020;37(4):699–726.

31. Pontén B. The fasciocutaneous flap: its use in soft tissue defects of the lower leg. Br J Plast Surg 1981;34(2):215–20.

32. Masquelet AC, Romana MC, Wolf G. Skin island flaps supplied by the vascular axis of the sensitive superficial nerves: anatomic study and clinical experience in the leg. Plast Reconstr Surg 1992; 89(6):1115–21.

33. Chang SM, Zhang F, Xu DC, Yu GR, Hou CL, Lineaweaver WC. Lateral retromalleolar perforator-based flap: anatomical study and preliminary clinical report for heel coverage. Plast Reconstr Surg 2007;120(3):697–704.

34. Kneser U, Bach AD, Polykandriotis E, Kopp J, Horch RE. Delayed reverse sural flap for staged reconstruction of the foot and lower leg. Plast Reconstr Surg 2005;116(7):1910–1917.2.

35. Baumeister SP, Spierer R, Erdmann D, Sweis R, Levin LS, Germann GK. A realistic complication analysis of 70 sural artery flaps in a multimorbid patient group. Plast Reconstr Surg 2003;112(1): 129–40. discussion 141-2.

Pediatrics

Foot Drop, Hindfoot Varus, and Tibialis Posterior Tendon Transfer in Cerebral Palsy

Lydia J. McKeithan, MD[a], Amanda T. Whitaker, MD[a,b],*

KEYWORDS

- Split tibialis posterior tendon transfer • Hindfoot varus • Footdrop • Cerebral palsy

KEY POINTS

- Tibialis posterior transfer is a successful surgery for hindfoot varus and foot drop in cerebral palsy with careful patient selection.
- The hindfoot must be flexible to inversion/eversion and ankle to dorsiflexion on the examination.
- Motion analysis should demonstrate swing phase activity of the tibialis posterior on electromyography if dorsiflexion is desired.
- The tibialis posterior transfer technique should be selected that best addresses the underlying deformity or deficiency

HISTORY OF TIBIALIS POSTERIOR TENDON TRANSFERS

Tendon transfers in the lower extremity have been performed for more than 100 years. Alessandro Codivilla (1851–1913), an Italian surgeon, is credited for the principles of tendon transfers, including the tibialis posterior through the interosseous membrane for foot drop. Tendon transfers were refined and optimized through the polio epidemic and upper extremity war injuries. In cerebral palsy, Duncan and colleagues first described a posterior tibialis tendon transfer to the dorsum of the foot.[1] Because of issues with overcorrection, Kaufer presented his study on the split tibialis posterior tendon transfer.[2] Since 1977, there have been refinements of the indications, surgical techniques, complications, and outcomes.

INDICATIONS

The classic indication for a tibialis posterior tendon transfer is a paralytic common peroneal nerve resulting in ankle equinus, hindfoot varus,-midfoot inversion, and foot dorp. The common peroneal nerve is the most commonly injured nerve in the lower extremity and is susceptible to injury due to its fixed position proximally at the pelvis and distally as it enters the anterior fascial compartment of the leg.[3–5] However, in cerebral palsy, abnormal nerve and muscle activity can result in varus deformity of the hindfoot and gait difficulties. Varus deformity of the hindfoot in cerebral palsy can be caused by the tibialis posterior, tibialis anterior, or both the tibialis posterior and tibialis anterior.[6] Given this complexity, the principles of tendon transfers, good physical evaluation, and proper surgical planning are needed as a foundation for appropriate patient selection (**Box 1**).

Principles of Tendon Transfer in Cerebral Palsy

There are several principles of tendon transfer surgery.[7] The muscle-tendon unit must be

a Department of Orthopaedic Surgery, University of California Davis, 4860 Y Street, Suite 3800, Sacramento, CA, USA; b Department of Orthopaedic Surgery, Shriners Children's Hospital Northern California, 2425 Stockton Boulevard, Sacramento, CA 95817, USA
* Corresponding author. Shriners Children's Hospital Northern California, 2425 Stockton Boulevard, Sacramento, CA 95817, USA
E-mail addresses: Amanda.Whitaker@shrinenet.org; atwhitaker@ucdavis.edu

Orthop Clin N Am 53 (2022) 311–317
https://doi.org/10.1016/j.ocl.2022.03.005
0030-5898/22/© 2022 Elsevier Inc. All rights reserved.

expendable and have other muscles with similar action. The tibialis posterior, flexor digitorum longus, flexor hallucis longus, and gastrocnemius-soleus complex all plantarflex and/or invert the hindfoot.[8] For ankle dorsiflexion and inversion, the tibialis anterior, extensor hallucis longus, and extensor digitorum longus have redundant activity. This redundant activity can be compromised due to abnormal muscle activity in cerebral palsy. Splitting the tendon decreases the potential for weakness and deformity overcorrection.

The transferred muscle must either have reasonable selective motor control or have activity in-phase with the pattern of the desired function. Selective motor control exists when the child can activate and control the muscle in isolation. The muscle also should be active in the gait cycle during the phase of desired activity of the transfer. This would be activity during the swing phase if dorsiflexionis desired with the tibialis posterior transfer. Children with cerebral palsy often have poor distal selective motor control, so for the tibialis posterior tendon to work as a dorsiflexor, it must have activity during the swing phase and not rely on selective motor control.[9,10]

Another principle of tendon transfers is that one grade of strength is lost after transfer. This can be due to friction or the force required to pull free of the surrounding scar tissue.[7,11] Another mechanism of strength lost after tendon transfer is overtensioning of the muscle. There could also be a lack of adaptation by the muscle and tendon to the stretch.[12] In cerebral palsy, there is no quantification of strength lost with tendon transfers in the lower extremity.[13,14]

The muscle and tendon to be transferred must have adequate expansion to act as a dynamic transfer. The tibialis posterior has the longest lever arm of the muslces around the foot and ankle. The next longest lever arm is the tibialis anterior. This long lever arm lends well to tendon transfers for pathologic inversion of the subtalar joint or hindfoot varus.[8] The proper tension of the muscle is not clear. Too much tension in the muscle and the sarcomeres will lengthen beyond their contractibility and be unable to generate force.[15] The muscles in children with cerebral palsy have a stiffer extracellular matrix, increased sarcomere length, fewer serial sarcomeres, and more fibrosis.[16,17] This difference in muscle architecture may decrease the amount of tension allowed for proper muscle contraction. Due to the inherent muscle stiffness, the tendon transfer may alternatively serve as a static transfer, or internal brace.[18] The joint should be positioned so the resting tension of the tendon transfer is neutral, or functional against gravity.[11]

The tendon must have a direct line of pull for the force to be appropriately distributed. An angle more than 45° will lose power due to friction.[11] The direction of the tendon will dictate how the tendon transfer will affect the joint, as a dorsal insertion will be more of an ankle dorsiflexor, and a lateral insertion will be more of a hindfoot evertor.

The path through which the tendon transfer travels must be a favorable environment, not prone to scar. A tissue bed of fat is ideal for the tendon to glide. A nonfavorable tissue bed is through an existing scar or a skin graft. This principle must be considered when transferring a tendon through the interosseus membrane. The path through the interosseus membrane must be large enough to allow the tendon to glide. In addition, the muscle needs enough strength and expansion to break free the scar tissue as it forms. This would support early mobilization of the joint after tendon transfer.

The joint at which the tendon transfer is intended to work must be flexible.[19] A dynamic or static tendon transfer will not correct stiff joints and bony deformity. Many articles have reported poor outcomes for tendon transfers with an undercorrected underlying deformity at the time of surgery. The subtalar and tibiotalar joints must have the desired passive range of motion prior to the tibialis posterior tendon transfer. If not, additional soft tissue procedures and possible skeletal realignment are required before tendon transfer.[20]

Motion analysis with fine-wire electromyography (EMG) is the gold standard for evaluating a foot drop, hindfoot varus, and potential tibialis posterior tendon transfer.[8] The tibialis posterior is responsible for early subtalar joint control. The tibialis posterior muscle is active in a typical gait pattern only during the stance phase. The peaks of muscle activation are at loading response and the middle of terminal stance, or the moment of contralateral foot contact. Ideal motion analysis data for tibialis posterior tendon transfer are tibialis posterior EMG activity during swing phase, a varus hindfoot, a plantarflexed foot in swing, and good strength and selective motor control of foot plantarflexion and inversion. For example, a child may have no tibialis anterior activity on EMG during swing phase or weakness on an examination with tibialis posterior EMG activity in swing phase. In this case, a tibialis posterior tendon transfer can prevent foot drop in swing, create dorsiflexion, and allow them to ambulate without a brace safely.

Tibialis posterior transfer improves foot drop, hindfoot varus, callus formation over the lateral border of the foot, fifth metatarsal stress fractures, prominence of the lateral malleolus, the need for swing phase bracing and decreases recurrent varus deformity in the correct patient. However, patient selection is paramount.

Physical Examination

The classic physical examination finding of an overactive posterior tibialis muscle, or weak dorsiflexors and evertors, is an equinovarus foot with limited active dorsiflexion and eversion. Essential components of the physical examination involve evaluating the range of motion, individual muscle strength, and selective motor control. The typical range of motion about the ankle and hindfoot is 20° of dorsiflexion, 50° of plantarflexion, 5 to 10° of inversion, and 5° of eversion. Dorsiflexion and plantarflexion are tested by having the patient sit on the edge of the table with their knees bent, allowing the gastrocnemius muscle to relax to eliminate the restriction of dorsiflexion. The examiner holds the calcaneus to stabilize the subtalar joint and has the forefoot inverted.

Inversion and eversion occur about the subtalar joint between the talocalcaneal, talonavicular, and calcaneocuboid joints. Inversion and eversion can be tested by having the patient remain seated with the examiner stabilizing the distal end of the tibia with one hand and gripping the calcaneus with the other. Inversion and eversion are tested by actively or passively moving the hindfoot.

The tibialis anterior is the predominant muscle for ankle dorsiflexion and contributes to inversionof the hindfoot. It inserts on the medial cuneiform and plantar first metatarsal base. Strength is tested with the patient sitting on the table's edge with their foot dorsiflexed and inverted. The examiner supports the distal leg with one hand and places their thumb on the dorsum of the foot. While pushing on the first metatarsal head, the examiner forces the foot into plantarflexion and eversion against resistance to measure anterior tibialis strength.

The tibialis posterior is the predominant muscle for foot inversion and has a minor role in foot plantarflexion.[21] It inserts on the navicular tubercle and medial cuneiform. Strength is tested by plantarflex and invert the foot against resistance. . The single-leg heel rise measures the functional strength of the tibialis posterior. The patient is asked to raise the opposite foot off the ground while balancing against a stable surface. Then the patient is asked to lift the heel and stand on their toes on the affected foot. Inability to raise the heel, lack of hindfoot inversion, or weakness indicate poor tibialis posterior strength.[22]

The Coleman block test is used to measure the flexibility of a hindfoot varus deformity.[23] For this test, the patient is asked to place their foot's heel and lateral border on a block with the first, second, and third metatarsals hanging freely. The patient then places their total weight onto the block as the first metatarsal is allowed to fall to the ground. If the heel falls into valgus or neutral, the varus deformity is considered flexible. .

The confusion test measures active ankle dorsiflexion. While sitting, the hip is flexed, the knee is bent, and resistance is added to the knee. A confusion test is considered positive when the tibialis anterior contracts when the patient is asked to flex their hip against resistance. The forefoo supinates and hindfoot transitions to varus in a flexible foot. A positive test suggests the tibialis anterior may play a role in the hindfoot deformity, but cannot predict walking kinematics. It is used widely in patients with cerebral palsy who may have a strong flexor pattern and limited ability to dorsiflex the ankle while the hip and knee are in an extension, an essential movement for gait.[24]

A good tibialis posterior tendon transfer candidate will have strong selective motor control and a flexible hindfoot varus on Coleman block testing. Examination findings that lead to a poor outcome after tibialis posterior transfer are a rigid hindfoot varus , poor muscle strength and poor selective motor control.

Motion Analysis

The tibialis posterior can contribute to hindfoot varus in both swing and stance phases or continuously throughout the gait cycle. The tibialis anterior can contribute to hindfoot varus in stance phase alone or cthroughout the gait cycle, but not if hindfoot varus is present in only swing phase.[6] If varus is in only stance phase, the muscle responsible is either the tibialis anterior or tibialis posterior, but not both.[6] Hindfoot varus typically occurs continuously in both swing and stance phases.[6] For this reason, the timing of hindfoot varus during the gait cycle often cannot determine the muscle imbalance. The muscle responsible for the dynamic hindfoot varus is identifiedthrough the timing of the tibialis anterior and posterior EMG related to the gait cycle. Tibialis anterior EMG can be obtained through a surface electrode; however, tibialis posterior EMG must be measured through fine-wire electrode into the muscle. It is essential to recognize that muscle activation does not change even with physical therapy after tendon transfer in cerebral palsy.[9] If a muscle is active only in stance phase, it will continue to be active only in stance phase and will not be retrained to be a swing phase muscle.

The kinematic assessment of hindfoot varus can be challenging to determine depending on the marker constructs used by the gait laboratory. Single-segment foot models are often used, correlating the foot's motion to the first metatarsal head, fifth metatarsal head, calcaneus, and the tibia. This can falsely represent the contribution of the hindfoot, midfoot, and forefoot to the observed varus deformity. Several multisegment foot models examine the dynamic state within the foot; however, they are technically challenging with higher variability between and within models.[26,27] Pedobarography will demonstrate increased lateral foot pressure and decreased pressure at the heel, most notably at initial contact.

SURGICAL TECHNIQUES

The ideal tibialis posterior tendon transfer surgical technique is determined based on the physical examination and motion analysis. In cerebral palsy, a split tendon transfer is preferred. Muscle spasticity leads to an overpull of the muscle in the direction

of the transfer, which will result in overcorrection of the deformity if the entire tendon is transferred.[9] By taking one-half of the tendon and leaving the other half at the insertion, the muscle can have a balanced force centered on the tendon limbs and have less recurrence or overcorrection.[9] Other procedures, such as gastrocnemius-soleus recession, Achilles lengthening, or osteotomies, are standard concomitant procedures due to the presence of additional deformities. An examination under anesthesia is critical to compare and confirm the passive range of motion of the foot and ankle.

The initial approach to the split tibialis posterior tendon transfer is well reported.[28] An incision is made over the tibialis posterior insertion, and half of the tendon is released. A nonabsorbable suture is placed in the released splittendon. Multiple incisions are made along the course of the tibialis posterior on the medial aspect to the musculotendinous junction, usually at the distal one-third to one-half of the tibia (Fig. 1). The tendon is passed posterior to the tibia and anterior to the neurovascular bundle. After the release and split of the tibialis posterior tendon, there are a variety of insertion locations and techniques described depending on the pre-operative weakness and deformity to correct.

The tibialis posterior can be passed through the interosseous membrane and inserted onto the lateral cuneiform.[28,29] This direction allows the tibialis posterior to act as a foot dorsiflexor. The tendon path through the interosseous membrane must be made wide enough that the tendon can easily glide with minimal scarring. The tendon can also be routed through the interosseus membrane and inserted into the peroneus brevis.[28,30] This position creates eversion of the hindfoot with some dorsiflexion. However, the route is less direct. It also changes the tendon insertion from a bone to atendon. If length is needed and the surgical plan is to insert

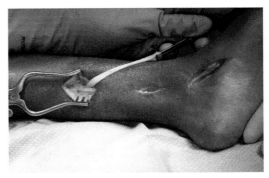

Fig. 1. Multiple medial incisions for releasing the split tibialis posterior tendon.

on the peroneus brevis, the dorsal half of the brevis can be split from the musculotendinous junction to the insertion, leaving the bony insertion intact. The split portion of the brevis can then be sutured to the split part of the tibialis posterior. One critique of this technique is scarring that may occur and bind the tendon transfer crossing the interosseus membrane.

Another path of the split posterior tibialis tendon transfer is around the lateral aspect of the fibula and inserted onto the peroneus brevis.[9,28,31,32] This direction of force acts as an evertor and weak plantarflexor, creating a neutral hindfoot position. The re-positioning to the peroneus brevis requires intact and strong tibialis anterior to dorsiflex the foot.

For those with combined tibialis posterior and tibialis anterior activity with the hindfoot varus in stance and swing, the tibialis anterior can be split and the posterior tibialis lengthened.[25,33] The split tibialis anterior can be routed to the cuboid for improved dorsiflexion, foot eversion, and neutral hindfoot position.[25,33] The peroneus brevis can also be split from the musculotendinous junction and sutured to the split tibialis anterior as described above.

The surgical challenges can be minimized with planning and technical pearls. An inflatable bump under the hip of the operative leg can assist with foot positioning to obtain access to the medial and lateral side without an assistant externally rotating the leg (Fig. 2).[34] To gain additional length for the tendon, the residual limbs (both medial and lateral) of split tibialis posterior tendon transfer can be lengthened with a Z-plasty.[32] Alternatively, the divided tendon can be resplit proximal to distal with a suture at the distal junction to prevent split propagation. Suture anchors can also add length to the transferred tendon into the bone.[35]

The traditional approach to insertion of the tibialis posterior onto the lateral cuneiform is a drill hole the diameter of the tendon into the lateral cuneiform, the tendon passing through to the plantar aspect of the foot affixed with a button.[29] Others have described drilling 2 holes and suturing the tendon onto itself.[33] Suture anchors and bioabsorbable screws can be used for bony fixation with higher pullout strength than the traditional tendon/bone interface in biomechanical studies.[35,36]

Postoperative care consists of casting for 6 weeks. Some brace for 6 months after casting.[29,33] Others determine if the transfer is working postoperatively via physical examination and prescribe a brace as needed.[31] Some allow weight-bearing immediately in the cast.[19,32] This variability in postoperative protocols may influence healing, muscle recovery, and outcomes after split tibialis posterior tendon transfers, however further well designed studies are required to determine the most effective postoperative treatment.

Poor outcomes have been described related to surgical technique when the entire posterior tibialis tendon is transferred or released in children with cerebral palsy, the transfer is combined with an Achilles overlengthening, or the skeletal deformity is not corrected.[19,30]

OUTCOMES AFTER TIBIALIS POSTERIOR TENDON TRANSFER IN CEREBRAL PALSY

Many studies have mixed results of tibialis posterior tendon transfers in cerebral palsy due to the lack of motion analysis and proper EMG. Moreover, many studies include rigid deformities of the foot and ankle that were not corrected during tendon transfer. Poor outcomes can be linked to a failure to identify ideal candidates for tibialis posterior transfer.[9,10,19,25] Incomplete correction due to fixed deformity will result in continued deformity. For example, the split

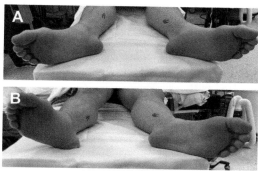
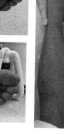
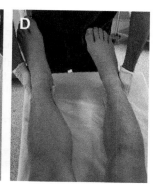

Fig. 2. Foot positioning with an inflatable bump.

tibialis posterior is transferred behind the tibia and inserted into the peroneus brevis, and the tibialis anterior is weak. In this case, the foot will continue to lack dorsiflexion strength and require an orthosis. Overcorrection can occur due to spasticity of the tibialis posterior muscle or overtensioning the transfer. The dynamic deformity can persist if the wrong tendon was transfered due to incomplete data lacking both tibialis anterior and posterior EMG . The tibialis posterior transfer can overcorrect the foot from equinovarus to calcaneovalgus if done when the patient is younger than 8 years old or the transfer is not a split transfer.[28,37]

SUMMARY

Children with cerebral palsy can present with hindfoot varus and difficulty clearing their foot in swing phase due to plantar flexion at the ankle. A thorough physical examination that includes passive and active range of motion with kinematics and dynamic EMG is critical in determining the cause of the deformity, the strong and redundant muscles, and the direction of force required to correct the deformity. A split tendon transfer is preferred to prevent overcorrection due to spasticity and the inability to reprogram muscle activity in cerebral palsy. A split tibialis posterior tendon transfer and soft tissue surgery will not correct a rigid deformity. Once the tibialis posterior has been identified as the deforming force or active during swing phase, it can be transferred to assist with dorsiflexion and eversion depending on the insertion site.

CLINICS CARE POINTS

- Tibialis posterior dysfunction contributes to most of the hindfoot varus in cerebral palsy, combined with tibialis anterior.
- Examine the strength and passive range of motion of the ankle and subtalar joint.
- Motionanalysis with fine-wire electromyography for the tibialis posterior is necessary for correct identification prior to transfer.
- Split the tendon in cerebral palsy to prevent overcorrection.
- For dorsiflexion assistance, transfer through the interosseus membrane.
- For eversion, transfer around the fibula.

DISCLOSURE

The authors have nothing to disclose.

REFERENCES

1. Gritzka TL, Staheli LT, Duncan WR. Posterior tibial tendon transfer through the interosseous membrane to correct equinovarus deformity in cerebral palsy. An initial experience. Clin Orthop 1972;89: 201–6.
2. Kaufer H. Split Tendon Transfer. Clin Orthop Relat Res 1977;128.
3. Katirji MB, Wilbourn AJ. Common peroneal mononeuropathy: a clinical and electrophysiologic study of 116 lesions. Neurology 1988;38(11):1723–8.
4. Aprile I, Caliandro P, La Torre G, et al. Multicenter study of peroneal mononeuropathy: clinical, neurophysiologic, and quality of life assessment. J Peripher Nerv Syst JPNS 2005;10(3):259–68.
5. Donovan A, Rosenberg ZS, Cavalcanti CF. MR imaging of entrapment neuropathies of the lower extremity. Part 2. The knee, leg, ankle, and foot. Radiogr Rev Publ Radiol Soc N Am Inc 2010;30(4):1001–19.
6. Michlitsch MG, Rethlefsen SA, Kay RM. The contributions of anterior and posterior tibialis dysfunction to varus foot deformity in patients with cerebral palsy. JBJS 2006;88(8).
7. White WL. Restoration of function and balance of the wrist and hand by tendon transfers. Surg Clin North Am 1960;40:427–59.
8. Perry J, Burnfield JM, editors. Gait analysis: normal and pathological function. 2nd edition. Thorofare, NJ: SLACK; 2010.
9. Green NE, Griffin PP, Shiavi R. Split posterior tibial-tendon transfer in spastic cerebral palsy. J Bone Joint Surg Am 1983;65(6):748–54.
10. Bisla RS, Louis HJ, Albano P. Transfer of tibialis posterior tendon in cerebral palsy. J Bone Joint Surg Am 1976;58(4):497–500.
11. OMER GEJR. Reconstructive procedures for extremities with peripheral nerve defects. Clin Orthop Relat Res 1982;163.
12. Takahashi M, Ward SR, Marchuk LL, et al. Asynchronous muscle and tendon adaptation after surgical tensioning procedures. J Bone Joint Surg Am 2010;92(3):664.
13. Jeng C, Myerson M. The uses of tendon transfers to correct paralytic deformity of the foot and ankle. Foot Ankle Clin 2004;9(2):319–37.
14. Das P, Kumar J, Karthikeyan G, et al. Peroneal strength as an indicator in selecting route of tibialis posterior transfer for foot drop correction in leprosy. Lepr Rev 2013;84(3):186–93.
15. Fridén J, Lieber RL. Evidence for muscle attachment at relatively long lengths in tendon transfer surgery. J Hand Surg 1998;23(1):105–10.

16. Smith LR, Lee KS, Ward SR, et al. Hamstring con- tractures in children with spastic cerebral palsy result from a stiffer extracellular matrix and increased in vivo sarcomere length. J Physiol 2011;589(Pt 10):2625–39.

17. Mathewson MA, Ward SR, Chambers HG, et al. High resolution muscle measurements provide in- sights into equinus contractures in patients with ce- rebral palsy. J Orthop Res Off Publ Orthop Res Soc 2015;33(1):33–9.

18. Dreher T, Wolf SI, Heitzmann D, et al. Tibialis pos- terior tendon transfer corrects the foot drop component of cavovarus foot deformity in Charcot-Marie-Tooth disease. J Bone Joint Surg Am 2014;96(6):456–62.

19. Root L, Miller SR, Kirz P. Posterior tibial-tendon transfer in patients with cerebral palsy. J Bone Joint Surg Am 1987;69(8):1133–9.

20. Davids JR. The foot and ankle in cerebral palsy. Orthop Manag Cereb Palsy 2010;41(4):579–93.

21. Myerson MS. Adult acquired flatfoot deformity. J Bone Jt Surg A 1996;78:780–92.

22. Johnson KA. Tibialis posterior tendon rupture. Clin Orthop 1983;177:140–7.

23. Coleman SS, Chesnut WJ. A simple test for hind- foot flexibility in the cavovarus foot. Clin Orthop 1977;123:60–2.

24. Davids JR, Holland WC, Sutherland DH. Signifi- cance of the confusion test in cerebral palsy. J Pediatr Orthop 1993;13(6):717–21.

25. Barnes MJ, Herring JA. Combined split anterior tibial-tendon transfer and intramuscular length- ening of the posterior tibial tendon. Results in pa- tients who have a varus deformity of the foot due to spastic cerebral palsy. J Bone Joint Surg Am 1991;73(5):734–8.

26. Schallig W, van den Noort JC, McCahill J, et al. Comparing the kinematic output of the Oxford and Rizzoli Foot Models during normal gait and voluntary pathological gait in healthy adults. Gait Posture 2020;82:126–32.

27. Di Marco R, Rossi S, Racic V, et al. Concurrent repeatability and reproducibility analyses of four marker placement protocols for the foot-ankle complex. J Biomech 2016;49(14):3168–76.

28. Flynn JM, Wiesel SW. Operative techniques in pe- diatric orthopaedics. Philadelphia, PA: Wolters Kluwer Health/Lippincott Williams & Wilkins; 2011.

29. Saji MJ, Upadhyay SS, Hsu LC, et al. Split tibialis posterior transfer for equinovarus deformity in ce- rebral palsy. Long-term results of a new surgical procedure. J Bone Joint Surg Br 1993;75(3): 498–501.

30. Mulier T, Moens P, Molenaers G, et al. Split poste- rior tibial tendon transfer through the interosseus membrane in spastic equinovarus deformity. Foot Ankle Int 1995;16(12):754–9.

31. Kling TF, Kaufer H, Hensinger RN. Split posterior tibial-tendon transfers in children with cerebral spastic paralysis and equinovarus deformity. J Bone Joint Surg Am 1985;67(2):186–94.

32. Aleksić M, Baščarevic Z, Stevanović V, et al. Modified split tendon transfer of posterior tibialis muscle in the treatment of spastic equinovarus foot deformity: long-term results and comparison with the standard procedure. Int Orthop 2020; 44(1):155–60.

33. Hoffer MM, Barakat G, Koffman M. 10-year follow- up of split anterior tibial tendon transfer in cerebral palsied patients with spastic equinovarus defor- mity. J Pediatr Orthop 1985;5(4):432–4.

34. Herzenberg JE. Inflatable bump to facilitate expo- sure during foot surgery. Foot Ankle 1992;13(1):42–3.

35. Fennell CW, Ballard JM, Pflaster DS, et al. Compar- ative evaluation of bone suture anchor to bone tun- nel fixation of tibialis anterior tendon in cadaveric cuboid bone: a biomechanical investigation. Foot Ankle Int 1995;16(10):641–5.

36. Núñez-Pereira S, Pacha-Vicente D, Llusá-Pérez M, et al. Tendon transfer fixation in the foot and ankle: a biomechanical study. Foot Ankle Int 2009;30(12): 1207–11.

37. Chang CH, Albarracin JP, Lipton GE, et al. Long- term follow-up of surgery for equinovarus foot deformity in children with cerebral palsy. J Pediatr Orthop 2002;22(6):792–9.

Hand and Wrist

Sagittal Band Injury and Extensor Tendon Realignment

Nicholas James, MD[a],*, Nolan Farrell, MD[b],
Benjamin Mauck, MD[b], James Calandruccio, MD[b]

KEYWORDS

- Sagittal band • Extensor tendon • Extensor tendon dislocation • Sagittal band reconstruction

KEY POINTS

- Injury to the sagittal band can cause pain, extensor tendon subluxation, or dislocation.
- Nonoperative treatment involves splinting the affected metacarpophalangeal (MCP) joint in extension within 3 weeks of injury.
- Direct surgical repair of the sagittal band can be performed if the tissue quality is adequate; if not, reconstruction needs to be considered.
- The use of local anesthetic and testing the stability of the tendon intraoperatively are important to obtain proper soft-tissue balancing.

INTRODUCTION

The sagittal bands are important structures that surround the metacarpal heads and metacarpophalangeal (MCP) joints that centralize the extensor digitorum communis (EDC), extensor indicis proprius (EIP), and extensor digiti minimi (EDM) tendons over each metacarpal head. Injury to the sagittal bands can cause pain, subluxation, or dislocation of the extensor tendons. These injuries can be caused by direct laceration of the sagittal bands or more commonly closed disruptions. The injury mechanism in the closed setting is generally a direct blow to the MCP joint, forceful resisted finger extension, or angular motions such as flicking.[1] Injury to the long finger is most common, likely due to the tendon's more superficial location and relatively loose fibrous attachment to the sagittal band compared with other fingers. Other predisposing factors include the more distal incorporation of the common extensor tendons into the extensor hood and more prominent oval shape of the extensor tendon at the level of the MCP joint.[2,3] Most of the injuries occur to the radial sagittal band with ulnar subluxation or dislocation of the tendon, although there are reports of ulnar-sided injury with radial dislocation.[4] In addition to the aforementioned features that increase the incidence of extensor tendon subluxation in the long finger, the radial digits have less robust juncturae, further increasing the likelihood of extensor tendon subluxation in these digits.[5] Rayan and Murray[6] classified sagittal band injuries into 3 types. Type I is an injury to the sagittal band, either contusion or partial tear without tendon subluxation. Type II involves injury to the sagittal band with subluxation of the extensor tendon. Type III involves injury to the sagittal band with dislocation of the extensor tendon.

[a] Editorial Campbell Clinic Foundation, 1211 Union Avenue, Suite 510, Memphis, TN 38104, USA; [b] Department of Orthopaedic Surgery and Biomedical Engineering, University of Tennessee Health Science Center - Campbell Clinic, 1211 Union Avenue, Suite 510, Memphis, TN 38104, USA
* Corresponding author.
E-mail address: nickjames484@gmail.com

Orthop Clin N Am 53 (2022) 319–325
https://doi.org/10.1016/j.ocl.2022.02.004
0030-5898/22/© 2022 Elsevier Inc. All rights reserved.

CLINICAL PRESENTATION AND DIAGNOSIS

Classically the diagnosis of sagittal band injuries is made clinically. The patient will often present with pain and swelling along the radial side of the affected MCP joint.[7] They may complain of a snapping sensation at the MCP joint with range of motion of the finger. Patients may have an extension deficit, particularly in Type III injuries.[8] However, if the finger is passively extended, the patient can maintain extension at the MCP joint, differentiating it from an extensor tendon rupture. There will often be a history of trauma, such as a direct blow to the MCP joint, but such an injury can also occur spontaneously with minimal to no trauma.[1] As mentioned previously the long finger is most often involved, although patients may present with multiple finger involvement, which is seen more commonly in rheumatoid arthritis.[9] Patients also may develop ulnar deviation of the digit due to the abnormal pull of the extensor tendon.[7,9] Plain radiographs are often normal but can be used to rule out MCP collateral ligament avulsion injuries. Ultrasound or MRI can be helpful if the patient has significant swelling and the clinical diagnosis is unclear. These tests may show subluxation or dislocation of the EDC tendon, or the underlying predispositions such as synovitis in inflammatory disorders (ie, systemic lupus erythematosus or rheumatoid arthritis).

ANATOMY

Extension of the fingers involves an intricate relationship between the extrinsic and intrinsic muscles of the forearm and hand. The extrinsic muscles originate proximal to the wrist crease and include the EDC, EIP, and EDM. The tendons pass deep to the extensor retinaculum in the fourth dorsal compartment, containing the EDC and EIP, and the fifth dorsal compartment, containing the EDM. On the dorsum of the hand, the extensor tendons are interconnected by the juncturae tendinum (**Fig. 1**). The juncturae tendinum functions to coordinate extension, stabilize the extensor tendons, and prevent complete independent digit extension.[10] The ulnar tendons generally have a greater number and more robust juncturae compared with the radial tendons.[5] In addition there are rarely juncturae connections to the EIP and occasionally no juncturae in the second intermetacarpal space between the index and long fingers.[5] The extensor tendons are tightly bound to the dorsum of the

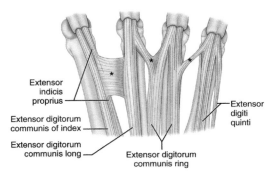

Extensor indicis proprius

Extensor digitorum communis of index

Extensor digitorum communis long

Extensor digiti quinti

Extensor digitorum communis ring

Fig. 1. A, Extensor tendons with connecting juncturae. (*Adapted from* Calandruccio JH. Extensor tendon injuries. In Azar FM, Beaty JH (eds.). *Campbell's Operative Orthopaedics*, 13th edition, Philadelphia, Elsevier, 2021, pp. 3388.)

MCP joint and the phalanges by an extensive retinacular system. At the level of the MCP joint, the extensor tendon enters the dorsal aponeurosis and is joined by the sagittal bands. The sagittal bands are made up of deep and superficial fibers that originate on the volar plate and intermetacarpal ligament and insert radially and ulnarly on the extensor tendon of each respective digit (**Fig. 2**) The sagittal bands function to maintain the alignment of the extensor tendon over the MCP joint, limit the proximal excursion of the extensor tendon, and prevent bowstringing.[11] The extrinsic extensor tendons course distally as the central slip, inserting on the dorsal base of the middle phalanx. A small portion of the common extensor tendon splits off radially and ulnarly proximal to the proximal interphalangeal joint and joins with and courses distally with the intrinsic tendons, inserting on the dorsal base of the distal phalanx as the terminal slip. The intrinsic tendons are the volar margins of the extensor apparatus and course distally dorsal to the rotational axis of the proximal interphalangeal (PIP) joint, and their radial and ulnar counterparts join to become the terminal slip, providing the extension of the PIP and the distal interphalangeal (DIP) joints.

MANAGEMENT

Nonoperative management is indicated for patients who present within 3 weeks of injury.[6,7,12] Treatment consists of a period of splinting the MCP in neutral or slight extension for 3 to 4 weeks. This can be performed with a static or dynamic splint such as a relative motion or yoke splint that keeps the affected MCP joint slightly extended, 25 to 35°, compared with the other digits.[6,8,12] The relative motion splint

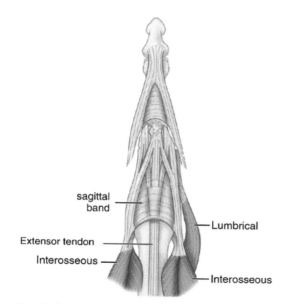

sagittal
band

Lumbrical

Extensor tendon

Interosseous

Interosseous

Fig. 2. Extensor mechanism with the sagittal bands over the metacarpal head. (*Adapted from* Calandruccio JH. Extensor tendon injuries. In Azar FM, Beaty JH (eds.). *Campbell's Operative Orthopaedics*, 13th edition, Philadelphia, Elsevier, 2021, pp. 3395.)

is designed to treat middle and ring finger injuries as the uninjured radial and ulnar digits are incorporated in the splint. After the immobilization period, patients may begin structured active range of motion exercises with intermittent splint wear between sessions and at night. Splinting is then discontinued at 6 to 8 weeks.[6–8]

Patients presenting later than 2 to 3 weeks or those who have failed to improve with splinting are candidates for surgical intervention. Surgical management includes direct repair or reconstruction of the sagittal band. Ideally, when operating on a sagittal band it should be performed with the patient under local anesthesia to confirm tendon stability through active range of motion before leaving the operating room. If the tissue quality is adequate, direct repair results in a good outcome.[1,2,6–8,13] Depending on the amount of scar tissue present, the release of the ulnar sagittal band or juncturae may be indicated.[6,14] If the residual tissue of the injured sagittal band is of poor quality, then reconstruction is indicated. There are many described techniques for reconstruction of the sagittal band. Most of the techniques involve using a slip of the EDC as a distally based graft and tethering it radially around the radial collateral ligament, lumbrical tendon, volar plate, or the deep transverse metacarpal ligament.[3,15–19]

SURGICAL GENERAL PRINCIPLES

In the acute setting, if there is adequate tissue, direct suture repair of the sagittal band, with or without the release of the contralateral aspect of the extensor structure, can yield adequate results.[1,2,6–8,13] Again, adequacy of the repair should be demonstrated intraoperatively. The EDC and EIP may need to be repaired directly to each other in instances of intrasubstance tearing and concomitant ulnar and radial subluxations.[7]

In reconstructive circumstances, extensor tendon centralization over the MP joint can be accomplished most easily with the use of distally based portions of the common or proper extensor tendons or their associated juncturae tendinae. A prerequisite for the stabilization of the soft-tissue component over the MP joint is the management of coexistent MP joint deformities. Subluxed or dislocated MP joints, as well as angular deformities of the metacarpal-forearm axis, should ideally be corrected before commencing to fine tune the extensor tendon instability about the MP joints. Moreover, radial collateral ligament instability in conjunction with common extensor tendon subluxation predisposes to a more difficult and less reliable stabilization procedure. Isolated common extensor tendon subluxation usually results from relatively minor traumatic forces and the foregoing provides a reliable way to correct such deformities.

All procedures for extensor tendon realignment are ideally performed with the patient under local anesthesia so that the patient can demonstrate the restoration of normal tendon mechanics through a full arc of digital flexion and extension. A field block well proximal to the planned dorsal skin incision and infiltration in the interdigital space on the side where the distal portion of the stabilization technique will be performed is preferred. A volar field block is avoided when possible to avoid intraoperative intrinsic paralysis.

Surgical Technique: Single-Digit Involvement
A 6.0-cm curved incision is made centered over the involved MP joint. The flap base is oriented to preserve the best possible important sensory innervated portions of the hand; thus, the index finger flap is based radially and the small finger-based ulnarly. Regardless of the incision chosen, all sensory branches are preserved as well as possible. This can be reliably achieved by initial dissection down to the venous and sensory nerve pathways in the valley between the adjacent metacarpal heads. Careful elevation of the skin flap over the involved metacarpal head from proximal to distal usually will reveal any sensory branches in the area.

Once the skin flap has been successfully raised, the reducibility of the tendon can be assessed. Radially directed traction on the extensor tendon at right angles to its longitudinal course should easily position the tendon over the midpoint of the metacarpal head. If the tendon cannot be easily reduced, then release of the ulnar deviating restraints is indicated before commencing with a radial-sided tendon tether procedure. Adhesion release between the sagittal band and the underlying MP joint capsule with a Freer elevator may suffice; however, if the tendon still cannot be easily reduced, gradual or complete sectioning of the ulnar sagittal band may be required. Sometimes the ulnar junctural communications may need to be released, and sections of this left attached to the common extensor tendon distally may be used for the reconstruction or augmentation of the final stabilization construct. Over-sectioning of the ulnar sagittal band is not advised unless absolutely necessary because an opposite instability pattern could ensue.

Once the common extensor tendon can be comfortably reduced over the midline of the MP joint, then either a junctural communication or a portion of the common or proper extensor tendon can be prepared to augment the deficient transverse fibers of the radial sagittal band. A 1.5-mm to 2.0-mm wide tendinous or junctural strip is dissected, beginning over the mid-portion of the metacarpal head and extending proximally to the level of the distal portion of the wrist extensor retinaculum (**Fig. 3**). Gentle traction before sectioning the tendon can significantly increase the length of the distally based tendon strip to a length of approximately 6.0 cm. This may also decrease the likelihood of the transected proximal end of the tendon/juncturá slip from being palpable about the extensor retinaculum. Should the remaining junctura on the side to which the tendon is subluxed or dislocated (usually ulnar) be a deforming force, then it should be transected after a portion of it is used for the reconstruction.

A single suture is placed to secure the distally based tendon strip at its origin over the mid-portion of the metacarpal head to prevent further tendon splitting distally (**Fig. 4**).

A mosquito hemostat or similar instrument is used to create a proximal-to-distal tunnel on the radial side of the MP joint through firm soft tissue extending just past the MP joint (**Fig. 5A, B**). This passageway may be through a portion of the radial collateral ligament and/or under the intermetacarpal ligament in the second through fourth web spaces. The precise

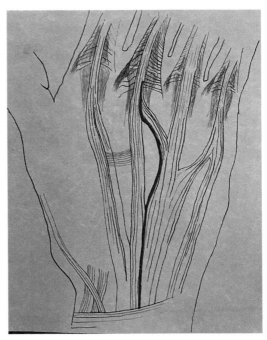

Fig. 3. Portion of junctura (*green line*) to be used for the reconstruction of an ulnar subluxation of middle finger.

location of this passageway is unimportant, but it needs to prevent the tendon/juncturá slip from migrating dorsally. The tendon strip is passed through this tunnel with the same instrument.

The lumbrical tendon is then identified on the volar radial side of the proximal phalangeal base and a pathway dissected around this tendon. The prepared slip is drawn under this lumbrical tendon and delivered to the reduced common extensor tendon (**Fig. 6**).

The prepared slip is passed through an opening in the reduced extensor tendon and secured with another single suture to keep the tendon centralized over the MP joint.

A tenodesis maneuver may be performed by passively flexing and extending the wrist to assess the alignment of the stabilized tendon; however, the preferred method is to have the patient gently extend and flex the finger fully to verify the desired tracking of the common extensor tendon. Alterations in the construct tension may be performed with reinforcing sutures to finalize the reconstruction before obtaining hemostasis and wound closure.

A volar forearm-based MP joint flexion block splint is then applied, and the patient is seen at 10 to 14 days for suture removal and initiation of a formalized therapy program.

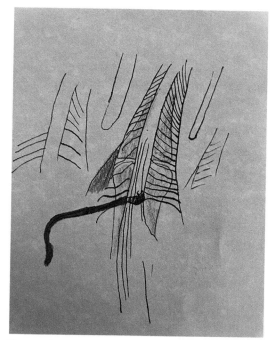

Fig. 4. The detached and distally based junctural slip is passed through the common extensor tendon at the midportion of the metacarpal head and anchored with a suture.

Surgical Technique: Multiple Digits

Attritional sagittal band laxity rheumatologic processes, such as rheumatoid arthritis and systemic lupus erythematosus, may predispose multiple fingers to extensor tendon subluxations. In such cases, all MP joints can be easily accessed through longitudinal incisions centered between the MP joints of the index-middle and the ring-small fingers. The distal extent of the incision should stop a few millimeters short of the web and course proximally about 4.5 cm in length.

The details for the reconstruction are similar to that described for a single-digit above; however, reconstruction for the index finger will require the use of a portion of either the EDC or EIP tendons as junctural communications to the index finger are structurally insignificant.

RECOVERY AND REHABILITATION

At 3 weeks active range of motion of the wrist is initiated. At 4 weeks the splint is the transition to a hand-based orthosis, and gentle digit flexion and full extension are begun, working up to a full active range of motion. At 6 weeks passive range of motion and light activities of daily living out of the orthosis are allowed. At 9 weeks the orthosis is discontinued, and by 10 to 12 weeks patients may resume normal activities without limitation.

OUTCOMES

Acute sagittal band injuries that are seen within 3 weeks of injury are treated nonoperatively, ideally 10 to 14 days, regardless of the grade of injury, generally yielding a good result.[6,7,12,20] Rayan and Murray[6] reported 18 patients treated nonoperatively in a static splint, 9 Type I, 3 Type II and 6 Type III. All patients but one (Type I injury) had complete resolution of pain. Catalano and colleagues[8] reported 11 Type III injuries treated for 8 weeks in a relative motion splint. Conservative treatment failed in 3 patients, one of whom was not compliant with splint wear and continued having painful subluxation of the tendon. In a series of 94 patients, Roh and colleagues[20] reported 71% success with nonoperative treatment in patients presenting within 7 weeks. Multivariable logistic analysis found that manual labor, longer symptom duration, and Type III injuries were associated with a

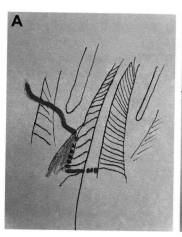

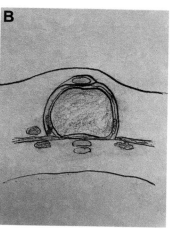

Fig. 5. (*A*) The junctural slip is channeled proximal to distal through firm soft tissue which will prevent the slip from migrating dorsally. (*B*) Cross-section about the metacarpal head, indicating the junctural slip either through or deep (*green dot*) to the collateral ligament.

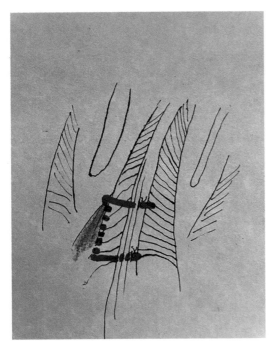

Fig. 6. The reconstruction is completed. The junctural slip is passed around the lumbrical tendon and drawn through a slit and sutured to in the centralized common extensor tendon.

higher likelihood of treatment failure, with the duration of symptoms greater than 3 weeks having the highest association with failure.[20]

In acute injuries with adequate tissue for repair, the result is generally good.[1,2,6–8,13] Ishizuki reported excellent results after repair of 16 sagittal band ruptures, with the resolution of pain and no recurrence of tendon instability.[1] A similar outcome was obtained by Inoue and Tamura who reported excellent results in 14 patients who underwent direct repair.[7] When tissue quality was poor and direct repair was not possible, reconstruction was indicated. The series was generally small, but the reported results of sagittal band reconstruction were good to excellent overall, with the resolution of pain and no recurrence of instability.[7,14,17,18,21,22] Watson and colleagues described a technique of using a distally based slip of the EDC tendon and looping it around the deep transverse ligament, recreating the radial sagittal band. The MP joint was immobilized with a Kirshner wire in 15 to 20° of flexion for 3 weeks. Good results were obtained in all 16 patients.[3] Shiode and Moritomo reported good results in 6 patients who underwent long finger EDC realignment by creating a tether using an ulnar slip of the index finger EDC tendon and weaving it through the long finger EDC tendon.[21] Kang and Carlson described a technique using palmaris longus autograft to create a pulley at the level of the metacarpal head, passing the graft through the metacarpal head and around the EDC tendon. They reported good results in 6 fingers with the resolution of pain and subluxation.[22]

These series did not experience any complications, though possible complications of both primary repair and reconstruction would be infection, joint stiffness, continued pain, or recurrent subluxation.

SUMMARY

The sagittal band is a vital component of the extensor component, and disruption can cause pain, subluxation, or dislocation of the extensor tendon. Patients seen within 3 weeks of injury can be treated conservatively with splinting followed by a gradual range of motion for 8 weeks. Surgical management is indicated in patients who present after 3 weeks or those in whom splinting has failed. If the tissue is of adequate quality, primary repair may be possible. If it is not, there are multiple reconstructive options including the one presented in this article that yield good results. We believe it is important to have the patients when possible perform a range of motion during the procedure to ensure proper balancing of the tendon.

CLINICS CARE POINTS

- Sagittal band injuries can be successfully treated within 3 weeks of injury with splinting.
- If tissue quality is adequate, primary repair of the sagittal band can be performed.
- If significant tension is required to align the extensor tendon, consider release of ulnar-sided scar tissue of the ulnar sagittal band.
- If tissue quality is poor, reconstruction of the sagittal band is required.
- Surgery should be performed with the patient under local anesthesia to ensure proper tendon alignment through an active range of motion.

DISCLOSURE

N. James - None, N. Farrell - None, B. Mauck - Olympus Endoscopy (outside of this work), J. Calandruccio- None.

REFERENCES

1. Ishizuki M. Traumatic and spontaneous dislocation of extensor tendon of the long finger. J Hand Surg Am 1990;15(6):967–72.
2. Kettelkamp DB, Flatt AE, Moulds R. Traumatic dislocation of the long-finger extensor tendon. a clinical, anatomical, and biomechanical study. J Bone Joint Surg Am 1971;53(2):229–40.
3. Watson HK, Weinzweig J, Guidera PM. Sagittal band reconstruction. J Hand Surg Am 1997;22(3): 452–6.
4. Ritts GD, Wood MB, Engber WD. Nonoperative treatment of traumatic dislocations of the extensor digitorum tendons in patients without rheumatoid disorders. J Hand Surg Am 1985;10(5):714–6.
5. von Schroeder HP, Botte MJ, Gellman H. Anatomy of the juncturae tendinum of the hand. J Hand Surg Am 1990;15(4):595–602.
6. Rayan GM, Murray D. Classification and treatment of closed sagittal band injuries. J Hand Surg Am 1994;19(4):590–4.
7. Inoue G, Tamura Y. Dislocation of the extensor tendons over the metacarpophalangeal joints. J Hand Surg Am 1996;21(3):464–9.
8. Catalano LW, Gupta S, Ragland R, et al. Closed treatment of nonrheumatoid extensor tendon dislocations at the metacarpophalangeal joint. J Hand Surg Am 2006;31(2):242–5.
9. Dell PC, Renfree KJ, Below Dell R. Surgical correction of extensor tendon subluxation and ulnar drift in the rheumatoid hand: long-term results. J Hand Surg Br 2001;26(6):560–4.
10. von Schroeder HP, Botte MJ. The functional significance of the long extensors and juncturae tendinum in finger extension. J Hand Surg Am 1993; 18(4):641–7.
11. Scott SC. Closed injuries to the extension mechanism of the digits. Hand Clin 2000;16(3):367–73, viii.
12. Araki S, Ohtani T, Tanaka T. Acute dislocation of the extensor digitorum communis tendon at the metacarpophalangeal joint. a report of five cases. J Bone Joint Surg Am 1987;69(4):616–9.
13. Arai K, Toh S, Nakahara K, et al. Treatment of soft tissue injuries to the dorsum of the metacarpophalangeal joint (Boxer's knuckle). J Hand Surg Br 2002;27(1):90–5.
14. Lee JH, Baek JH, Lee JS. A reconstructive stabilization technique for nontraumatic or chronic traumatic extensor tendon subluxation. J Hand Surg Am 2017;42(1):e61–5.
15. Takahashi N, Iba K, Hanaka M, et al. Sagittal band reconstruction in the index finger using a modified Elson technique. J Orthop Surg (Hong Kong) 2018; 26(1). 2309499017749985.
16. Kilgore ES, Graham WP, Newmeyer WL, et al. Correction of ulnar subluxation of the extensor communis. Hand 1975;7(3):272–4.
17. Carroll C, Moore JR, Weiland AJ. Posttraumatic ulnar subluxation of the extensor tendons: a reconstructive technique. J Hand Surg Am 1987;12(2): 227–31.
18. Vyrva O, Kvann J, Karpinsky M, et al. A reconstructive extensor tendon centralization technique for sagittal band disruption. Tech Hand Up Extrem Surg 2020;24(1):20–5.
19. ElMaraghy AW, Pennings A. Metacarpophalangeal joint extensor tendon subluxation: a reconstructive stabilization technique. J Hand Surg Am 2013;38(3): 578–82.
20. Roh YH, Hong SW, Gong HS, et al. Prognostic factors for nonsurgically treated sagittal band injuries of the metacarpophalangeal joint. J Hand Surg Am 2019;44(10):897.e1–5. e5.
21. Shiode R, Moritomo H. Tether creation between the second and third extensor digitorum communis for third extensor tendon subluxation at the metacarpophalangeal joint. Tech Hand Up Extrem Surg 2018;22(4):146–9.
22. Kang L, Carlson MG. Extensor tendon centralization at the metacarpophalangeal joint: surgical technique. J Hand Surg Am 2010;35(7):1194–7.

Shoulder and Elbow

Remplissage for Anterior Shoulder Instability
History, Indications, and Outcomes

William Polio, MD, Tyler J. Brolin, MD*

KEYWORDS

- Remplissage • Hill-Sachs • Glenoid track • Subcritical glenoid bone loss

---

KEY POINTS

- A Hill-Sachs lesion is an impaction fracture of the posterolateral humeral head articular surface that may increase a patient's risk of recurrent instability.
- Calculation of the glenoid track and Hill-Sachs interval allows surgeons to predict preoperatively engagement of the Hill-Sachs lesion with the anterior glenoid rim.
- Remplissage is a posterior capsulodesis and infraspinatus tenodesis used to fill the Hill-Sachs defect, converting the lesion to extra-articular as well as decreasing anterior humeral head translation.
- The addition of remplissage to Bankart repair in patients with off-track Hill-Sachs lesions, subcritical glenoid bone loss, or the young contact athlete decreases recurrent instability rates and improves patient-reported outcomes.

INTRODUCTION

The shoulder is the most frequently dislocated large joint due to the unique anatomic architecture and lack of bony architectural support. The low level of constraint and high degree of mobility of the shoulder provides a large arc of motion but presupposes the joint to instability. Males are 2.5 times more likely than females to sustain a dislocation, with a peak incidence between age 20 and 29 years and a majority occurring during sports or recreational activities.[1] Traumatic glenohumeral instability is associated with compromise of one or several static and/or dynamic stabilizers. Static stability of the glenohumeral joint is conferred via the bony architecture, negative intra-articular pressure, glenoid labrum, glenohumeral ligaments, and the coracohumeral ligament, whereas dynamic stabilizers include the rotator cuff, deltoid, long head of the biceps, and scapulothoracic musculature. Most cases of traumatic unilateral anterior instability result in disruption of the anteroinferior capsulolabral complex as well as an impaction fracture of the humeral head or Hill-Sachs lesion. Bankart lesions have an incidence of 78% in acute first-time dislocations and 97% in cases of recurrent instability, whereas Hill-Sachs lesion has an incidence of 65% in acute first-time dislocations and 93% in cases of recurrent instability (**Tables 1 and 2**)[2].

Historically, management of anterior shoulder instability in North America has been arthroscopic or open Bankart repair. Success of this procedure is well documented and is predicated on restoring the native anteroinferior labral "bumper" as well as tensioning the anterior band of the inferior glenohumeral ligament. However, Burkhart and De Beer[3] in 2000 first highlighted the role of bony defects of either the glenoid or humeral head in recurrent shoulder instability. The investigators defined significant glenoid bone loss as an inverted pear geometry of the glenoid, which corresponds to

---

Department of Orthopaedic Surgery and Biomedical Engineering, University of Tennessee-Campbell Clinic, Memphis, TN, USA

* Corresponding author. 1211 Union Avenue, Suite 510 Memphis, TN 38104.

E-mail address: tbrolin@campbellclinic.com

Table 1		
Anterior instability categories		
Group	**Glenoid Defect**	**Hill-Sachs Lesion**
1	<25%	On track
2	<25%	Off track
3	≥25%	On track
4	≥25%	Off track

From Di Giacomo G, Itoi E, Burkhart SS. Evolving concept of bipolar bone loss and the Hill-Sachs lesion: from "engaging/non-engaging" lesion to "on-track/off-track" lesion. Arthroscopy 2014;30(1):90–8. doi:10.1016/j.arthro.2013.10.004.

greater than or equal to 25% inferior glenoid bone loss. Significant humeral head bone loss was described as a lesion engaging with the anterior rim of the glenoid. Using these criteria, the rates of recurrent dislocation following isolated arthroscopic Bankart repair were 67% in the setting of significant bone loss, compared with 4% without significant bone loss.[3] Given the most common complication following isolated anterior labral repair is recurrent instability, it is imperative that surgeons identify risk factors for recurrent shoulder instability such as glenoid or humeral head bone loss and formulate a surgical plan to mitigate these risks without jeopardizing patient function.[4] Recurrent instability rates following arthroscopic Bankart repair have been reported to be 8.5%,[5] whereas in contact athletes the recurrence rate increases to 17.8%.[6]

There is no consensus as to what value constitutes "critical" bone loss, which would necessitate conversion to bony augmentation procedure. Traditional values in the literature range from

Table 2	
Treatment paradigm	
Group	**Recommended Treatment**
1	Arthroscopic Bankart repair
2	Arthroscopic Bankart repair
3	plus remplissage
4	Latarjet procedure
	Latarjet procedure with or without humeral-sided procedure (humeral bone graft or remplissage), depending on engagement of Hill-Sachs lesion after Latarjet procedure

From Di Giacomo G, Itoi E, Burkhart SS. Evolving concept of bipolar bone loss and the Hill-Sachs lesion: from "engaging/non-engaging" lesion to "on-track/off-track" lesion. Arthroscopy 2014;30(1):90–8. doi:10.1016/j.arthro.2013.10.004.

20% to 27%.[7–9] More recently, interest has been shown in the role of subcritical bone loss to functional outcomes and risk of recurrence following standard Bankart repair. In a cadaveric model, creation of a 15% glenoid defect decreased the mean contact area in the anterior inferior quadrant by nearly 30% and increased the mean contact pressure by 75% with the arm in 60° abduction and 90° external rotation.[10] In finite element modeling, Klemt and colleagues[11] showed a high risk of dislocation during activities of daily living following Bankart repair with anterior glenoid defects of 16%. Shin and colleagues[12] followed 169 patients for 2 years following Bankart repair and found 17.3% glenoid bone loss to be predictive of failure, with 43% of patients sustaining recurrent instability events with bone loss above the threshold compared with 3.7% with bone loss below the threshold. Postoperative Single Assessment Numeric Evaluation (SANE) and American Shoulder and Elbow Surgeons (ASES) scores were also significantly higher in patients with less than 17.3% glenoid bone loss.[12] Shaha and colleagues[7] evaluated 73 consecutive Bankart repairs in a military population and found glenoid bone loss of 13.5% or more to be associated with poor clinical outcomes as assessed by Western Ontario Shoulder Instability (WOSI) score, even in patients without recurrent instability. Humeral head bone loss as low as 12.5% to 25% has been shown to lead to decreased anterior translation before dislocation, resulting in higher dislocation rates in a cadaveric study.[13] Bipolar bone loss further compromises glenohumeral stability following Bankart repair. In a biomechanical study, a medium-sized Hill-Sachs defect (1.47 cm^3) was created based on the 50th percentile lesion size on the computed tomographic (CT) scans of 142 patients with recurrent instability. A medium-sized Hill-Sachs defect was found to lead to compromise of Bankart repair in the presence of a glenoid bone defect as low as 8%.[14]

Bone block procedures or "arthroscopic plus" procedures, such as remplissage, have been suggested in lieu of standard Bankart repair for patients at high risk of recurrent instability. The use of Latarjet procedure for critical glenoid bone loss of 20% to 25% is well established; however, the ideal treatment of subcritical glenoid bone loss is not clearly defined. Remplissage has been suggested as an adjunct to Bankart repair in patients with subcritical glenoid bone loss and an "off-track" Hill-Sachs lesion. However, controversy still exists on whether to treat these types of injuries with Bankart repair in isolation or combined with remplissage versus with Latarjet. Young male athletes, particularly contact athletes, also represent a population at increased risk of recurrent instability following standard Bankart repair, with some investigators advocating for primary treatment with the addition of remplissage or Latarjet. The purpose of this article is to describe the development of remplissage and its techniques, as well as report indications and outcomes based on the degree of bone loss and sport participation.

Development of Remplissage

Flower[15] was the first to report on the presence of a groove excavated posterior to the greater tuberosity on the articular surface of the humeral head in his cadaveric dissections in 1861. Case reports of humeral head resections in the treatment of chronic or habitual shoulder dislocation between 1880 and 1903 further characterized the excavation of the posterior articular surface as the "typical lesion." Later, the lesion was named after Hill and Sachs, who in 1940 defined the lesion as an impaction fracture resulting in a flattening or groove on the posterolateral articular surface above the anatomic neck with a sharp line of increased density running along the medial border and floor of the groove parallel to the axis of the humerus. The investigators also first described its mechanism as due to posterolateral impingement of the humeral head on the glenoid rim in the abducted, externally rotated shoulder.[16] Connolly,[17] in 1972, was the first to describe the concept of filling in a Hill-Sachs lesion, with open transfer of the infraspinatus tendon, analogous to the already developed McLaughlin procedure for chronic posterior dislocations; this provided a dynamic checkrein to anterior humeral head gliding and converted the Hill-Sachs lesion into an extra-articular structure in an effort to prevent the defect from translating over the anterior glenoid rim.[17] Since that time, numerous other strategies have been suggested for treating Hill-Sachs lesion associated with recurrent dislocations, including open capsular shift to limit abduction and external rotation, osteochondral allograft transplantation, partial resurfacing, and transhumeral head plasty to elevate the impacted fracture.[18–20] The most widely used technique today is remplissage, which is a French term meaning "to fill." Wolf and Pollack,[18] in 2004, first described the arthroscopic remplissage technique, which involved a posterior capsulodesis and infraspinatus tenodesis to fill in the humeral head defect. The tenodesis converts the Hill-Sachs defect to extra-articular lesion and the posterior capsulodesis decreases anterior humeral head translation, both of which serve

to prevent engagement of the humeral head with the anterior glenoid rim. The arthroscopic remplissage is an adjunct procedure usually performed in conjunction with an arthroscopic Bankart repair.[18]

Evaluation of Hill-Sachs Lesions: The Glenoid Track

Although multiple classification systems have been developed for grading Hill-Sachs lesions based on size, none have been shown to guide or predict surgical treatment. More helpful for determining significance is the concept of the glenoid track, as originally described by Yamamoto and colleagues[21] in 2007. In a cadaveric study, they determined the glenohumeral contact area at varying levels of shoulder abduction with maximal external rotation and horizontal extension to determine the track the glenoid makes when contacting the humeral head. The findings were then correlated to live patients based on CT 3D reconstruction (3D recon). The glenoid track was found to shift from the inferomedial to superolateral aspect of the posterior humeral articular surface. On average, the glenoid track extends 18.4 mm medial to the insertion of the rotator cuff on the greater tuberosity, which corresponds to 84% of the glenoid width. The results of this study are useful for determining whether a Hill-Sachs lesion will or will not engage with the anterior glenoid rim. An engaging Hill-Sachs lesion would be considered "off track," meaning the medial aspect of the Hill-Sachs lesion will override the glenoid rim and risk dislocation. In contrast, an "on-track" Hill-Sachs lesion remains in articulation with the face of the glenoid with articulating bone adjacent to the defect and should not engage by overhanging the glenoid rim. Thus, the location is more important than the length or depth of the Hill-Sachs lesion, because medial lesions are more likely to be considered "off track." The size of the glenoid track depends on the width of the glenoid, therefore any bone loss on the anterior glenoid rim will narrow the glenoid track and increase the likelihood of an off track, engaging Hill-Sachs lesion and recurrent instability.[21]

In the setting of bipolar bone loss, quantification of the glenoid track before surgery will provide more accurate assessment of the contribution of bone loss to instability. Before the concept of glenoid track, dynamic arthroscopic examination was used to determine engagement of a Hill-Sachs lesion. Typically, this was done before Bankart repair to prevent excess stress placed on the repair by placing the arm in abduction and external rotation. However, capsulolabral repair alters the anatomic and biomechanical context of the shoulder such that the likelihood of engagement of a Hill-Sachs lesion decreases.[22] Kurokawa and colleagues[25] defined the "true engaging Hill-Sachs lesion" as either a lesion that engages after Bankart repair or a lesion that extends over the glenoid track. True engaging Hill-Sachs lesions were overestimated using dynamic arthroscopic assessment before Bankart repair (34%–46%),[23,24] with a prevalence rate likely more near 7%.[25] Di Giacomo and colleagues[22] provides a technique for reliably determining the glenoid track in relation to the Hill-Sachs lesion based on direct arthroscopic measurement or CT 3D recon with humeral and scapular subtraction sequences. Using CT 3D recon with humeral subtraction, the glenoid is viewed en face and the size of bony defect, if present, is estimated. Numerous techniques are available, including defect length, width to length ratio, glenoid index, and the Pico method; however, the investigators suggested the use of the contralateral shoulder as a reference.[22] The side-to-side differences in glenoid area have been shown to average 1.8%.[26] The greatest horizontal diameter width of the glenoid D on both shoulders is measured and the size of the defect d is measured by subtracting uninvolved from involved glenoid. The humeral head is then evaluated on the CT 3D recon with scapula retraction. The medial margin of the footprint of the rotator cuff and Hill-Sachs lesion is identified. Next, a line measuring 83% of the glenoid width is placed extending from the medial margin of the rotator cuff footprint. This line represents the glenoid track if there is no bone loss on the glenoid. If a bone defect is present, the value d is subtracted from this 83% line to set the medial edge of the glenoid track. If the Hill-Sachs lesion is located within the boundary of this line, it is considered "on track," whereas if the Hill-Sachs extends over the line it is considered "off track." Oftentimes, a bone bridge exists between the lateral margin of the Hill-Sachs lesion and the rotator cuff attachment. The combined width of the bone bridge and Hill-Sachs lesion represents the Hill-Sachs interval (HSI), whose medial margin is the critical point in determining on-track versus off-track status. A summary of authors' technique can be found in **Box 1** and **Fig. 1**, along with their proposed treatment algorithm in the setting of bipolar bone loss.[22]

Gyftopoulos and colleagues[27] evaluated the feasibility of determining on-off track status of

---

Box 1
How to determine whether Hill-Sachs lesion is "on track" or "off track"

- Measure the diameter (D) of the inferior glenoid either by arthroscopy or from 3D CT scan
- Determine the width of the anterior glenoid bone loss (d).
- Calculate the width of the glenoid track (GT) by the following formula: GT = 0.83 D−d.
- Calculate the width of the HSI, which is the width of the Hill-Sachs Lesion (H) plus the width of the bone bridge (BB) between the rotator cuff attachments and the lateral aspect of the Hill-Sachs Lesion: HSI = HS + BB.
- If HSI is greater than GT, the HS is off track, or engaging. If HSI is less than the HS is on track, or nonengaging.

From Di Giacomo G, Itoi E, Burkhart SS. Evolving concept of bipolar bone loss and the Hill-Sachs lesion: from "engaging/non-engaging" lesion to "on-track/off-track" lesion. Arthroscopy 2014;30(1):90–8. doi:10.1016/j.arthro.2013.10.004.

---

a Hill-Sachs lesion with MRI. The glenoid bone loss was determined using the circle-of-best-fit technique, and the glenoid track width was determined using the above-described formula 0.83 D-d. MRI prediction of track status was compared with arthroscopic findings of engagement. Overall, MRI accuracy was found to be 84%, with a positive predictive value of 65% and negative predictive value of 91%.[27] An example of calculating the glenoid track and Hill-Sachs interval using MRI can be found in **Fig. 2**.

Di Giacomo and colleagues[28] developed the glenoid track instability management score (GTIMS), which sought to incorporate the concept of glenoid track into the instability injury severity score (ISIS). Balg and Boileau described the ISIS as a 10-point scale based on preoperative risk factors of age ($\leq$20 = 2 points [pts]), degrees (competitive = 2 pts) and type (contact/overhead = 1 pt) of sports participation, shoulder hyperlaxity (1 pt), presence of a Hill-Sachs lesion on anteroposterior (AP) external rotation radiograph (2 pts), and loss of contour of the glenoid on AP radiographs (2 pts). A score of greater than 6 was reported to have a 70% risk of instability after arthroscopic Bankart repair, causing the investigators to advocate for a Bristow-Latarjet procedure in these patients.[29]

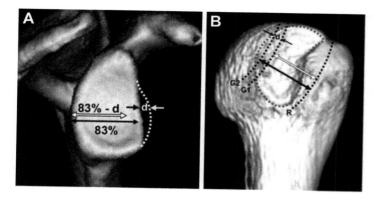

Fig. 1. Case with bony defect of glenoid (A) and large Hill-Sachs lesion (B). By use of the contralateral glenoid as a reference (100%), 83% width is determined (*black double-headed arrow*). Then the defect width (D) is subtracted from this 83% length to obtain the glenoid track width for this case (*white double-headed arrow*). Dotted line R represents the medial margin of the rotator cuff attachments. It should be noted there is normally an intact bone bridge between the cuff attachments and the lateral border of the Hill-Sachs lesion. Dotted line G1 indicates the location of the medial margin of the glenoid track. If there had been no glenoid bony defect, the medial margin of the glenoid track would have been dotted line G2. In this case the Hill-Sachs lesion extends medially beyond the medial margin of the glenoid track (*dotted line* G1), so this is an off-track lesion.

Subsequently, Phadnis and colleagues[30] have validated the ISIS as a preoperative tool and reported a 70% risk of recurrence following Bankart repair in patients scoring greater than or equal to 4. Using a cutoff value of 4 for recommendation of a Latarjet procedure, the GTIMS allocates points the same way as ISIS for all criteria except for imaging. The GTIMS replaces the AP radiograph scores of ISIS to incorporate on-off track lesions status evaluated by CT 3D recons. A score of 4 is given for off-track lesions, whereas a score of 0 is given for on-track lesions. The investigators found that use of the GTIMS resulted in a significantly more conservative treatment algorithm, recommending Bankart repair in 85% of cases compared with 31% when using the ISIS. The overall rate of recurrent instability after Bankart repair was 8% following the GTIMS versus 4.5% following ISIS. The investigators believe that incorporating CT 3D recon imaging to determine the glenoid track helped avoid overestimating clinically irrelevant bone loss, thereby preventing some patient's from undergoing an open bone block procedure.[30]

In clinical practice, the use of the glenoid track can be difficult. CT scans remain the most accurate imaging modality for detecting osseus lesions and quantifying bone loss; however, many patients undergo MRI before referral. In addition, CT 3D recon with humeral and scapular retraction is preferred for the most accurate assessment of the glenoid track, rather than 2D assessment on MRI or CT. In most instances, contralateral shoulder imaging is not available for comparing the size of the native glenoid with the affected glenoid, which has led to the development of circle-of-best-fit measurements based on the intact posterior and inferior glenoid rims. This technique is more accurate on CT 3D recon, but MRI has been found to have moderate agreement. MRI may be advantageous when determining the Hill-Sachs interval, because the footprint of the rotator cuff is more accurately visualized.[31]

The evaluation of patient with anterior shoulder instability begins with a thorough history and physical examination. Patients with unilateral instability often describe a traumatic event

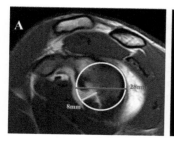
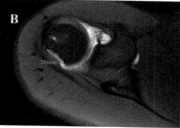

Fig. 2. (A) Sagittal T1-weighted magnetic resonance (MR) arthrogram showing anterior inferior glenoid bone loss. The red line estimates the intact glenoid diameter (28 mm). The yellow line indicates the amount of bone loss (8 mm). The glenoid track is 15.3 mm. (B) Axial fat-suppressed T2-weighted MR arthrogram showing a Hill-Sachs lesion measuring 20 mm, without a significant bone bridge. Because the Hill-Sachs interval is greater than the glenoid track, this lesion is defined as off-track.

resulting in their first dislocation, often with the arm in the abducted and externally rotated position. As structural damage becomes more extensive, dislocations can become more frequent and atraumatic. Special attention should be paid to the patient's age and their age at the time of the first dislocation, number of dislocations, mechanism of dislocation, activity level, and sport involvement. The presence of confounding medical conditions, such as seizures or chronic alcohol use, needs to be considered when developing a treatment plan. Physical examination should begin with inspection for atrophy and scapular winging, as well as palpation to determine areas of tenderness. Range-of-motion testing should be gentle and not beyond the range of apprehension to avoid iatrogenic dislocations. Rotator cuff and deltoid strength should be assessed, in addition to a thorough neurologic examination for the entire involved extremity. Numerous maneuvers have been described to evaluate anterior instability. Anterior apprehension testing is performed by bringing the arm to 90° abduction and 90° external rotation. If the patient experiences apprehension of impending dislocation the test is positive. Relocation testing is positive if the patient's apprehension is relieved by a posteriorly directed force on the anterior humeral head. The combination of apprehension and relocation testing has a specificity of 90.2% and sensitivity of 64.6%.[32] Load and shift testing is performed with the arm in 60° abduction and forward flexion. The humeral head is loaded onto the glenoid fossa and then shifted anterior and inferior while the scapula is stabilized. The results are graded as 0, minimal displacement; 1, translation to glenoid rim; 2, translation over glenoid rim with spontaneous relocation; and 3, translation over glenoid rim without spontaneous relocation. The specificity has been found to be 90% to 100% and sensitivity up to 71%.[33] The anterior drawer test is performed by shifting the humeral head anteriorly on the glenoid fossa and is considered positive if the patient experiences a sense instability with affected shoulder compared with the contralateral shoulder. The presence of a sulcus sign and calculation of Beighton score should also be evaluated to screen for patients with hyperlaxity. Standard radiographs should be obtained to confirm that the shoulder is currently reduced and to evaluate for fracture. Standard views include a Grashey, scapular Y, and axillary lateral views. Special radiographs to consider are the Stryker notch view, which is particularly helpful to evaluate Hill-Sachs lesions, as well as West Point axillary view for evaluation of the anteroinferior glenoid rim. The presence of bone loss on plain radiographs is an indication for advanced imaging with CT 3D recon or MRI (**Fig. 3**).

Remplissage Technique

Multiple techniques exist for the arthroscopic Hill-Sachs remplissage procedure. The procedure is analogous to arthroscopic repair of an articular-sided partial-thickness rotator cuff tear. The infraspinatus tendon and posterior capsule are fixated to the Hill-Sachs lesion. In general, techniques are distinguished by knotted or knotless fixation, subacromial or intra-articular viewing, and mattress versus pulley configuration. Wolf and Pollack[18] described a knotted horizontal mattress repair tied over 2 anchors in a mattress configuration. The investigators described glenohumeral joint viewing of the Hill-Sachs defect during anchor placement while tying the knots in the subacromial space.[18] In an effort to avoid tissue strangulation by engaging a larger footprint of the infraspinatus, Burkhart and colleagues, developed a subacromial knotted double pulley repair between 2 anchors. This technique involves viewing from the subacromial space for suture passing and knot tying.[34]

The authors' preferred technique is a knotless double pulley repair given the concern over symptomatic knots in the subacromial space. The patient is positioned in the lateral decubitus position using a bean bag. The arm is suspended by 6.75 kg traction in 45° of abduction with a slightly posterior line of pull. A posterior portal is established just inferior to the posterolateral acromial edge. Next, as in all standard labral repairs, an anteroinferior portal is established under needle localization just superior to the subscapularis tendon, ensuring the trajectory allows for anchor placement at the 5:30 position. A cannula is placed because this will serve as the working portal for suture passage and anchor placement for the Bankart repair. Finally, an anterosuperior portal is established just lateral and inferior to the acromioclavicular (AC) joint, entering the joint just behind the long head of the biceps tendon; this will serve as the viewing portal for the labral repair and remplissage procedure. The arthroscope is transitioned to the anterosuperior position and a cannula is placed in the posterior portal, which will serve as a retrieving portal for the Bankart repair as well as the working portal for the remplissage procedure. It is important to assess trajectory and location before cannula placement, which will aid in the later remplissage

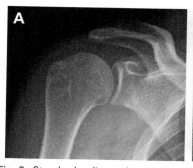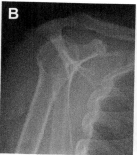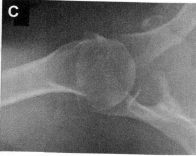

Fig. 3. Standard radiographs including Grashey (*A*), scapular Y (*B*), and axillary lateral (*C*) views demonstrating the Hill-Sachs lesion and anterior glenoid bone loss. This patient was sent for CT 3D recon with scapular and humeral subtraction for evaluation of bipolar bone loss and surgical planning.

technique. After the Bankart repair is completed the posterior cannula is backed slowly outside the joint and superficial to the capsule and infraspinatus tendon into the subacromial space; this is a check to ensure smooth motion of the cannula while visualizing the posterior capsule and infraspinatus tendon. A sharp trochar is advanced into the cannula and pierces the infraspinatus and capsule at the desired location for an inferior anchor in the Hill-Sachs defect, typically 5 mm from the articular surface and at the inferior extent of the Hill-Sachs lesion. For most procedures, Arthrex PEEK 2.9 Knotless Corkscrew anchors, Arthrex, Inc. Naples, FL are used. A second anchor is placed in a similar manner through the same posterior cannula at the superior extent of the Hill-Sachs lesion. It is imperative to keep track of each suture set from the individual anchors, which is accomplished using a hemostat, as well as limit unnecessary anterior force on the humeral head, which could disrupt the Bankart repair. To complete the remplissage, the repair suture of each anchor is then passed into the locking mechanism of the other anchor and is tensioned together at the same time to compress the tendon to bone. Arthroscopic images demonstrating this technique can be found in **Fig. 4.** Biomechanical testing has been performed comparing the knotted pulley technique to the knotless remplissage technique, which demonstrated higher load to failure of the knotless repair.[35]

Indications and Outcomes
The most common indication for remplissage is in the treatment of an "off-track" Hill-Sachs lesion with minimal glenoid bone loss. Franceschi and colleagues conducted a comparative study between 25 patients treated with arthroscopic Bankart repair alone and 25 patients treated with arthroscopic Bankart repair plus double-pulley remplissage. All patients had off-track Hill-Sachs lesions with an average size of 30% of the radius of the humerus, and importantly 11 patients (5 in the remplissage and 6 in Bankart-only group) had an anterior glenoid bone defect, averaging approximately 15%. At 2-year follow-up, the remplissage group had no episodes of recurrent instability, whereas the Bankart repair-alone group had a recurrence rate of 20%.[36] Hughes and colleagues compared Bankart repair with or without remplissage in the high-risk adolescent population with Hill-Sachs lesions and found that the addition of remplissage significantly decreased recurrence rates (13% versus 47%), while maintaining similar range of motion and patient outcome scores.[37] Buza and colleagues performed a systematic review that included 167 patients with a Hill-Sachs lesion treated with arthroscopic Bankart repair and remplissage. The investigators reported a 5.4% recurrence rate, a statistically nonsignificant loss of 3° of external rotation, and average postoperative Rowe score of 87.[38]

Subcritical glenoid bone loss is increasingly being recognized as a risk factor for recurrent instability following Bankart repair, and controversy exists as to the optimal treatment. Glenoid bone loss as low as 13.5% in an active population has been shown to be associated with inferior clinical outcomes following standard Bankart repair.[7] Biomechanical evidence suggests that remplissage can stabilize bipolar lesions with Hill-Sachs defects up to 30% and glenoid defects up to 17%.[39] A survey of 26 surgeons involved in the MOON shoulder group found that the addition of remplissage to Bankart repair was used most commonly for Hill-Sachs lesions measuring 11% to 20% or glenoid defects measuring 11% to 20%.[40] MacDonald and colleagues conducted a randomized controlled trial of 108 patients with an "off-track" Hill-Sachs lesion and glenoid

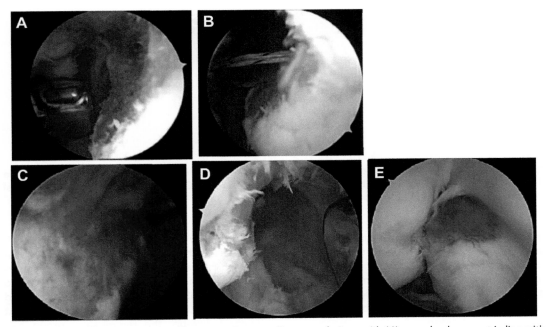

Fig. 4. Case 1: Arthroscopic images demonstrating remplissage technique with (A) cannula placement in line with desired location for an anchor followed by decortication and (B) placement of anchors. Case 2: (C) Hill-Sachs lesion followed by (D) decortication and (E) filling defect with remplissage.

bone loss less than 15% treated with Bankart repair or Bankart repair plus remplissage. The average Hill-Sachs lesion was 15% of the humeral head. The investigators found an 18% recurrence rate in the nonremplissage group compared with 4% in the remplissage group at 24 months. The odds ratio of recurrent instability in the nonremplissage group relative to the remplissage group was 5.49. This odds ratio increased to 11.5 if a large Hill-Sachs lesion was present (>15% humeral head or >20 mm).[41] A review of 5 comparison studies between arthroscopic Bankart repair alone versus arthroscopic Bankart repair plus remplissage in the setting a subcritical bone loss showed decreased recurrent instability rates in the remplissage group. The Bankart repair groups had recurrence rates ranging from 6.7% to 57%, whereas the Bankart plus remplissage group maintained recurrence rates between 0% and 20%. The addition of remplissage to Bankart repair reduced the odds ratio for recurrence between 0.07 and 0.88.[42]

Biomechanical data suggest that both remplissage and Latarjet effectively reduced the frequency of dislocation without consistently altering joint stiffness in a 25% Hill-Sachs model with intact glenoid rim, indicating either procedure may be appropriate treatment.[43] Among

MOON shoulder surgeons, the factors most predictive of patients undergoing Latarjet procedure were those involved in a high-risk sport, presence of glenoid bone loss 11% to 30%, and those undergoing revision surgery.[40] Yang and colleagues[42] compared remplissage versus Latarjet in 189 patients with subcritical glenoid bone loss and off-track Hill-Sachs lesion. No differences were found in revision rates or episodes of recurrent instability; however, the complication rate in the Latarjet group was significantly higher than that in remplissage, 12.1% versus 1%. No differences were found in patient-reported outcome measures in WOSI or SANE. In multivariate analysis, the odds of recurrent instability in the remplissage group were higher than those in the Latarjet group in patients with previous instability surgery (3.56), collision and contact athletes (2.37), those with 10% to 15% glenoid bone loss (1.28), and those with greater than 15% glenoid bone loss (6.48).[44] Cho and colleagues[45] compared the results of 37 patients who underwent Bankart repair and remplissage with 35 patients who underwent Latarjet in the setting of subclinical glenoid bone loss (average 8%–9%) and an engaging Hill-Sachs lesion. There was no significant difference in regard to recurrence rate (5.4% versus 5.7%), visual analog scale (VAS) score, Rowe score, or range of motion. There was a significant difference in regard to complication rate, 14.3% in Latarjet and 0% in remplissage.[45] Haroun and colleagues[46] performed a meta-analysis of 4 studies with 379 patients with subcritical glenoid bone loss (<20%) and either Hill-Sachs lesions sized greater than 20% to 30% or "off track." Patients either underwent treatment with Latarjet (185 patients) or Bankart repair and remplissage (194 patients). No difference was found in terms of recurrence rate (7% Latarjet vs 10% remplissage), patient outcome scores including VAS and Rowe score, or range of motion. The complication rate of Latarjet was significantly higher than that of remplissage, 9% versus 1%.[46]

Contact athletes, particularly among young males, represent a unique population that is known to be at higher risk of failure following standard Bankart repair. Yamamoto found that contact athletes had a recurrence rate 3 times that of noncontact athletes following arthroscopic Bankart repair.[47] Castagna and colleagues found following Bankart repair in adolescent contact and overhead athletes that the rate of failure was 21%, with 81% returning to their preinjury level of sport.[48] Some investigators argue that contact athletes may benefit from bone block procedures or more secure soft tissue procedures, such as remplissage, in the primary setting. Among all types of athletes, remplissage has been shown to have an excellent return to sport rate at 95%, with 81% returning to their preinjury level. Return rates were less encouraging in overhead-throwing athletes at 51% with 65% reporting continued problems with throwing.[49] A review of 77 American football and rugby patients with an average age 20 years and a Hill-Sachs lesion with glenoid bone loss less than 25% treated with remplissage found a recurrence rate of 5% with a 92% return to play rate at 7 months. Average Rowe score was 96 and SSV 92.[50] Domos and colleagues[51] compared outcomes in professional contact athletes with nonengaging Hill-Sachs lesions and minimal glenoid bone loss following Bankart repair with or without additional remplissage. The investigators found that the remplissage group had significantly lower recurrence rate (5% vs 30%) and reoperation rate (5% vs 35%), with similar return to play rates (100% vs 90%).[51] Some surgeons are still more likely to perform Latarjet than remplissage for high-risk athletes, regardless of glenoid bone loss.[40] Arciero and colleagues found that in contact athletes with subcritical bone loss, Latarjet had better WOSI scores (138 vs 231) and lower recurrence rate (30% vs 0%) than remplissage.[44]

Concern exists that remplissage may induce changes in shoulder biomechanics, such as range of motion or strength, due to the nonanatomic reduction of the infraspinatus into the Hill-Sachs defect. Merolla and colleagues[52] compared glenohumeral range of motion in 61 shoulders treated with arthroscopic Bankart repair and remplissage with the nonoperative shoulder, as well as 40 healthy controls. Loss of 9° of external rotation with the arm at the side was found in the operative cohort between the postoperative and nonoperative shoulders. None of the patients reported functional impairment due to the reduced external rotation. Significantly lower external rotation both with the arm at the side (68 vs 89°) and in 90° of abduction (74 vs 89°), as well as internal rotation in 90° of abduction (71 vs 81°), was found between the operative shoulder and healthy controls. No significant differences between any groups were found in regard to infraspinatus strength.[52] In a systematic review, an average loss of 9 to 14° of external rotation was found in 5 of 9 articles.[42] Ding and colleagues[53] investigated the postoperative features of the glenohumeral cartilage, range of motion, and anchor placement following remplissage in 21 patients with postoperative MRIs performed a minimum 2 years following surgery. A significant loss of external rotation (>15°) was found in 12 patients, which was positively correlated with significantly higher signal intensity of cartilage on the posterior humeral head. The investigators concluded that post-remplissage limitations in external rotation are correlated, at least partially, with relatively medial anchor placement (ie, an overly medial Hill-Sachs lesion). The recognition of a relatively medial Hill-Sachs lesion and its correlation to decreased external rotation should be especially recognized when considering remplissage in overhead athletes.[53] Some concern also exists that the tenodesis may also cause inflammation in the rotator cuff, which may lead to increased rates of subacromial decompression and glenohumeral debridement in the remplissage group.[44]

SUMMARY

Higher rates of recurrent glenohumeral instability following Bankart repair can be seen in the setting of bipolar bone loss and in young contact athletes. The glenoid track can account for bipolar bone loss to accurately predict engagement of Hill-Sachs lesions with the glenoid rim. Remplissage is a capsulotenodesis of the infraspinatus tendon that has been developed to address engaging, or "off-track," Hill-Sachs lesions. The addition of remplissage to Bankart repair has shown promising reductions in recurrent instability rates for patients with "off-track" Hill-Sachs lesions, subcritical glenoid bone loss, and contact athletes. Concerns exist for the nonanatomic nature of the procedure; however only mild reductions in external rotation have been shown, whereas strength and patient reported outcome data have been excellent.

CLINICS CARE POINTS

- The glenoid track can be calculated as GT = 0.83D-d, where D is the horizontal diameter of the intact glenoid and d is the width of glenoid bone loss

- The Hill-Sachs interval can be calculated as HSI= HS + BB, where HS is the width of the Hill-Sachs lesion and BB is the bone bridge between the lateral edge of the Hill-Sachs and the attachment of the rotator cuff

- If HSI is greater than GT, the Hill-Sachs lesion is "off track" or engaging, and consideration should be given to arthroscopic remplissage

- Biomechanical testing comparing the knotted pulley technique to knotless remplissage showed significantly higher loading forces required to displace the knotless repair compared with knotted, along with a higher load to failure of knotless repair

- A randomized controlled trial comparing patients treated with Bankart repair with or without remplissage in the setting of an engaging Hill-Sachs lesion and glenoid bone loss less than 15% showed an 18% recurrence rate in the nonremplissage group compared with 4% in the remplissage group.

- In the setting of primary shoulder instability with subcritical glenoid bone loss (<15%), arthroscopic remplissage has a similar rate of recurrent instability to Latarjet procedure with lower complication rates.

- A review of professional contact athletes with nonengaging Hill-Sachs lesions and minimal glenoid bone loss showed lower recurrence rates (5% vs 30%) with the addition of remplissage to Bankart repair, with a 100% return to sport rate in the remplissage group.

- In a systematic review, an average loss of 9° to 14° of external rotation was found following arthroscopic remplissage

---

DISCLOSURE

W. Polio: has nothing to disclose. T.J. Brolin: American Shoulder and Elbow Surgeons, board or committee member; Arthrex, paid consultant and research support; DJ Orthopaedics, research support; Elsevier, publishing royalties, financial or material support; Orthofix, Inc, research support; Orthopedic Clinics of North America, editorial or governing board.

REFERENCES

1. Zacchilli MA, Owens BD. Epidemiology of shoulder dislocations presenting to emergency departments in the United States. J Bone Joint Surg Am 2010; 92(3):542–9.
2. Yiannakopoulos CK, Mataragas E, Antonogiannakis E. A comparison of the spectrum of intra-articular lesions in acute and chronic anterior shoulder instability. Arthroscopy 2007;23(9): 985–90.
3. Burkhart SS, De Beer JF. Traumatic glenohumeral bone defects and their relationship to failure of arthroscopic Bankart repairs: significance of the inverted-pear glenoid and the humeral engaging Hill-Sachs lesion. Arthroscopy 2000; 16(7):677–94.
4. Wiesel BB, Gartsman GM, Press CM, et al. What went wrong and what was done about it: pitfalls in the treatment of common shoulder surgery. J Bone Joint Surg Am 2013;95(22):2061–70.
5. Harris JD, Gupta AK, Mall NA, et al. Long-term outcomes after Bankart shoulder stabilization. Arthroscopy 2013;29(5):920–33.
6. Leroux TS, Saltzman BM, Meyer M, et al. The influence of evidence-based surgical indications and techniques on failure rates after arthroscopic shoulder stabilization in the contact or collision athlete with anterior shoulder instability. Am J Sports Med 2017;45(5):1218–25.
7. Shaha JS, Cook JB, Song DJ, et al. Redefining "critical" bone loss in shoulder instability: functional outcomes worsen with "subcritical" bone loss. Am J Sports Med 2015;43(7):1719–25.
8. Beran MC, Donaldson CT, Bishop JY. Treatment of chronic glenoid defects in the setting of recurrent anterior shoulder instability: a systematic review. J Shoulder Elbow Surg 2010;19(5):769–80.
9. LU Bigliani, Newton PM, Steinmann SP, et al. Glenoid rim lesions associated with recurrent anterior dislocation of the shoulder. Am J Sports Med 1998;26(1):41–5.
10. Ghodadra N, Gupta A, Romeo AA, et al. Normalization of glenohumeral articular contact pressures after Latarjet or iliac crest bone-grafting. J Bone Joint Surg Am 2010;92(6):1478–89.

11. Klemt C, Toderita D, Nolte D, et al. The critical size of a defect in the glenoid causing anterior instability of the shoulder after a Bankart repair, under physiological joint loading. Bone Joint J 2019;101-B(1):68–74.

12. Shin SJ, Kim RG, Jeon YS, et al. Critical value of anterior glenoid bone loss that leads to recurrent glenohumeral instability after arthroscopic bankart repair. Am J Sports Med 2017;45(9):1975–81.

13. Sekiya JK, Wickwire AC, Stehle JH, et al. Hill-Sachs defects and repair using osteoarticular allograft transplantation: biomechanical analysis using a joint compression model. Am J Sports Med 2009; 37(12):2459–66.

14. Arciero RA, Parrino A, Bernhardson AS, et al. The effect of a combined glenoid and Hill-Sachs defect on glenohumeral stability: a biomechanical cadaveric study using 3-dimensional modeling of 142 patients. Am J Sports Med 2015;43(6):1422–9.

15. Flower WH. On pathologic changes produced in the shoulder joint by traumatic dislocation. Trans Path Soc Lond 1861;12:179–201.

16. Hill HA, Sachs MD. The grooved defect of the humeral head. a frequently underrecognized complication of dislocations of the shoulder joint. Radiology 1940;35:690–700.

17. Connolly J. Humeral Head defects associated with shoulder dislocations. Instr Course Lect 1972;12: 42045.

18. Wolf EM, Pollack ME. Hill-Sach's "Remplissage:" an arthroscopic solution for the engaging Hill-Sachs lesion. Arthroscopy 2004;20(Suppl 1):e14–5.

19. Chapovsky F, Kelly JDIV. Osteochondral allograft transplantation for treatment of glenohumeral instability. Arthroscopy 2005;21:1007.e1-4.

20. Re P, Gallo RA, Richmond JC. Transhumeral head plasty for large Hill-Sachs lesions. Arthroscopy 2006;22:798–798.e1. e4.

21. Yamamoto N, Itoi E, Abe H, et al. Contact between the glenoid and the humeral head in abduction, external rotation, and horizontal extension: a new concept of glenoid track. J Shoulder Elbow Surg 2007;16(5):649–56.

22. Di Giacomo G, Itoi E, Burkhart SS. Evolving concept of bipolar bone loss and the Hill-Sachs lesion: from "engaging/non-engaging" lesion to "on-track/off-track" lesion. Arthroscopy 2014; 30(1):90–8.

23. Cho SH, Cho NS, Rhee YG. Preoperative analysis of the Hill-Sachs lesion in anterior shoulder instability: How to predict engagement of the lesion. Am J Sports Med 2011;39:2389–95.

24. Zhu YM, Lu Y, Zhang J, et al. Arthroscopic bankart repair combined with remplissage technique for the treatment of anterior shoulder instability with engaging hill-sachs lesion: a report of 49 cases with a minimum 2- year follow-up. Am J Sports Med 2011;39:1640–7.

25. Kurokawa D, Yamamoto N, Nagamoto H, et al. The prevalence of a large Hill-Sachs lesion that needs to be treated. J Shoulder Elbow Surg 2013;22:1285–9.

26. Jeske HC, Oberthaler M, Klingensmith M, et al. Normal glenoid rim anatomy and the reliability of shoulder instability measurements based on intra-site correlation. Surg Radiol Anat 2009;31:623–5.

27. Gyftopoulos S, Beltran LS, Bookman J, et al. MRI evaluation of bipolar bone loss using the on-track off-track method: a feasibility study. AJR Am J Roentgenol 2015;205(4):848–52.

28. Di Giacomo G, Peebles LA, Pugliese M, et al. Glenoid track instability management score: radiographic modification of the instability severity index score. Arthroscopy 2020;36(1):56–67.

29. Balg F, Boileau P. The instability severity index score. a simple pre-operative score to select patients for arthroscopic or open shoulder stabilisation. J Bone Joint Surg Br 2007;89:1470–7.

30. Phadnis J, Arnold C, Elmorsy A, et al. Utility of the instability severity index score in predicting failure after arthroscopic anterior stabilization of the shoulder. Am J Sports Med 2015;43:1983–8.

31. Kwong CA, Gusnowski EM, Tam KK, et al. Assessment of bone loss in anterior shoulder instability. AOJ 2017;2(11).

32. Farber AJ, Castillo R, Clough M, Bahk M, McFarland EG. Clinical assessment of three common tests for traumatic anterior shoulder instability. J Bone Joint Surg Am. 2006;88(7):1467–74.

33. van Kampen DA, van den Berg T, van der Woude HJ, Castelein RM, Terwee CB, Willems WJ. Diagnostic value of patient characteristics, history, and six clinical tests for traumatic anterior shoulder instability. J Shoulder Elbow Surg 2013;22(10):1310–9.

34. Koo SS, Burkhart SS, Ochoa E. Arthroscopic double-pulley remplissage technique for engaging Hill-Sachs lesions in anterior shoulder instability repairs. Arthroscopy 2009;25(11):1343–8.

35. Funakoshi T, Hartzler R, Stewien E, Burkhart S. Remplissage Using Interconnected Knotless Anchors: Superior Biomechanical Properties to a Knotted Technique? Arthroscopy 2018;34(11): 2954–9.

36. Franceschi F, Papalia R, Rizzello G, Franceschetti E, Del Buono A, Panascì M, Maffulli N, Denaro V. Remplissage repair–new frontiers in the prevention of recurrent shoulder instability: a 2-year follow-up comparative study. Am J Sports Med 2012;40(11): 2462–9.

37. Hughes JL, Bastrom T, Pennock AT, Edmonds EW. Arthroscopic Bankart Repairs With and Without Remplissage in Recurrent Adolescent Anterior Shoulder Instability With Hill-Sachs Deformity.

Orthop J Sports Med 2018;6(12). 2325967118813981.

38. Buza JA 3rd, Iyengar JJ, Anakwenze OA, Ahmad CS, Levine WN. Arthroscopic Hill-Sachs remplissage: a systematic review. J Bone Joint Surg Am. 2014;96(7):549–55.

39. Garcia GH, Degen RM, Bui CNH, McGarry MH, Lee TQ, Dines JS. Biomechanical comparison of acute Hill-Sachs reduction with remplissage to treat complex anterior instability. J Shoulder Elbow Surg 2017;26:1088–96.

40. Bishop JY, Hidden KA, Jones GL, Hettrich CM, Wolf BR, MOON Shoulder Group. Factors Influencing Surgeon's Choice of Procedure for Anterior Shoulder Instability: A Multicenter Prospective Cohort Study. Arthroscopy 2019;35(7):2014–25.

41. MacDonald P, McRae S, Old J, Marsh J, Dubberley J, Stranges G, Koenig J, Leiter J, Mascarenhas R, Prabhakar S, Sasyniuk T, Lapner P. Arthroscopic Bankart repair with and without arthroscopic infraspinatus remplissage in anterior shoulder instability with a Hill-Sachs defect: a randomized controlled trial. J Shoulder Elbow Surg 2021;30(6):1288–98.

42. Liu JN, Gowd AK, Garcia GH, Cvetanovich GL, Cabarcas BC, Verma NN. Recurrence Rate of Instability After Remplissage for Treatment of Traumatic Anterior Shoulder Instability: A Systematic Review in Treatment of Subcritical Glenoid Bone Loss. Arthroscopy 2018.

43. Degen RM, Giles JW, Johnson JA, Athwal GS. Remplissage versus Latarjet for engaging Hill-Sachs defects without substantial glenoid bone loss: a biomechanical comparison. Clin Orthop Relat Res. 2014;472(8):2363–71.

44. Yang JS, Mehran N, Mazzocca AD, Pearl ML, Chen VW, Arciero RA. Remplissage Versus Modified Latarjet for Off-Track Hill-Sachs Lesions With Subcritical Glenoid Bone Loss. Am J Sports Med 2018;46(8):1885–91.

45. Cho NS, Yoo JH, Rhee YG. Management of an engaging Hill-Sachs lesion: arthroscopic remplissage with Bankart repair versus Latarjet procedure. Knee Surg Sports Traumatol Arthrosc 2016;24(12):3793–800.

46. Haroun HK, Sobhy MH, Abdelrahman AA. Arthroscopic Bankart repair with remplissage versus Latarjet procedure for management of engaging Hill-Sachs lesions with subcritical glenoid bone loss in traumatic anterior shoulder instability: a systematic review and meta-analysis. J Shoulder Elbow Surg 2020;29(10):2163–74.

47. Yamamoto N, Kijima H, Nagamoto H, Kurokawa D, Takahashi H, Sano H, Itoi E. Outcome of Bankart repair in contact versus non-contact athletes. Orthop Traumatol Surg Res. 2015;101(4):415–9.

48. Castagna A, Delle Rose G, Borroni M, Cillis BD, Conti M, Garofalo R, Ferguson D, Portinaro N. Arthroscopic stabilization of the shoulder in adolescent athletes participating in overhead or contact sports. Arthroscopy 2012;28(3):309–15.

49. Garcia GH, Wu HH, Liu JN, Huffman GR, Kelly JD 4th. Outcomes of the Remplissage Procedure and Its Effects on Return to Sports: Average 5-Year Follow-up. Am J Sports Med. 2016;44(5):1124–30.

50. Hoshika S, Sugaya H, Takahashi N, Matsuki K, Tokai M, Morioka T, Ueda Y, Hamada H, Takeuchi Y. Arthroscopic Soft Tissue Stabilization With Selective Augmentations for Traumatic Anterior Shoulder Instability in Competitive Collision Athletes. Am J Sports Med 2021;49(6):1604–11.

51. Domos P, Ascione F, Wallace AL. Arthroscopic Bankart repair with remplissage for non-engaging Hill-Sachs lesion in professional collision athletes. Shoulder Elbow 2019;11(1):17–25.

52. Merolla G, Paladini P, Di Napoli G, Campi F, Porcellini G. Outcomes of arthroscopic Hill-Sachs remplissage and anterior Bankart repair: a retrospective controlled study including ultrasound evaluation of posterior capsulotenodesis and infraspinatus strength assessment. Am J Sports Med 2015.

53. Ding Z, Cong S, Xie Y, Feng S, Chen S, Chen J. Location of the Suture Anchor in Hill-Sachs Lesion Could Influence Glenohumeral Cartilage Quality and Limit Range of Motion After Arthroscopic Bankart Repair and Remplissage. Am J Sports Med 2020;48(11):2628–37.

Soft Tissue Management in Shoulder Arthroplasty

Brandon Anthony Romero, MD, John Gabriel Horneff III, MD*

KEYWORDS

- Shoulder arthroplasty • Soft tissue • Rotator cuff • Reverse • Subscapularis repair

KEY POINTS

- A functional rotator cuff is essential to allow for a proper fulcrum to exist in the anatomic shoulder joint and allow for shoulder motion.
- The subscapularis tendon is traditionally taken down during exposure for shoulder arthroplasty. Options for taking down the tendon include tenotomy, osteotomy of the lesser tuberosity, and tendon peel off the tuberosity.
- Management of the long head of the biceps tendon is typically at the surgeon's discretion with tenotomy or tenodesis being the most common options for treatment.
- Proper capsular release in shoulder arthroplasty is beneficial for surgical exposure during the procedure and for improved range of motion postoperatively.

INTRODUCTION

The field of shoulder arthroplasty continues to grow, as the aging population has demanded more procedures to be performed every year.[1] As such, techniques are unceasingly being updated to improve patient function and implant longevity. Although the radiographically visible aspects of shoulder arthroplasty like bone cuts and implant position are important, they only make up half of the formula for a good arthroplasty. Meticulous attention to soft tissue management is an integral factor for a successful shoulder replacement.

THE ROTATOR CUFF

Much of the soft tissue techniques in shoulder arthroplasty revolve around the rotator cuff. The muscles of the rotator cuff serve important roles as mobilizers and dynamic stabilizers of the shoulder. Knowledge of the integrity and function of the patient's cuff muscles are vital for surgical planning and the success of total shoulder arthroplasty (TSA).

Biomechanics and Mechanism of Failure in Anatomic Total Shoulder Arthroplasty

The native shoulder requires a stable fulcrum for function. For a stable fulcrum to exist, the force couples made up of the cuff muscles and deltoid must be balanced. An intact anterior cuff balances the posterior cuff and vice versa, preventing imbalance in the transverse plane. The medially directed pull of inferior portion of the rotator cuff acts as a balance against the superiorly directed pull of the deltoid in the coronal plane. When a large cuff tear is present, the force couples are disrupted, leading to loss of the stable fulcrum and failure of function.[2] In its most significant form, this disruption presents with proximal migration of the humerus and pseudoparalysis of the arm (Fig. 1).

In anatomic shoulder arthroplasty, a rotator cuff tear can lead to disruption of force couples and translation of the humeral head during movement of the shoulder. When the humeral head is not centered in the glenoid, there is an increased amount of force applied to the edges of the polyethylene glenoid component. This often leads to an increased rate of polyethylene

University of Pennsylvania, 3737 Market Street 6th Floor, Philadelphia, PA 19104, USA
* Corresponding author.
E-mail address: jghorneff3@gmail.com

Orthop Clin N Am 53 (2022) 339–347
https://doi.org/10.1016/j.ocl.2022.02.001
0030-5898/22/© 2022 Elsevier Inc. All rights reserved.

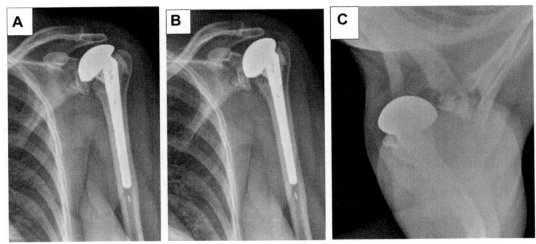

Fig. 1. Anatomic total shoulder arthroplasty after rotator cuff failure. Note the anterior and superior subluxation, as well as lucency around both the glenoid component and the humeral cement mantle. Shown are the Grashey (A), AP (B), and axillary (C) radiographs.

wear as well as loosening of the glenoid component. The repeated edge-loading of the polyethylene causes the polyethylene to tip in the direction of the loaded segment, ultimately causing glenoid loosening and failure, an occurrence dubbed the "rocking horse" phenomenon.[3] Because of the potential for this complication, success of the anatomic TSA hinges on the integrity of the rotator cuff.

The Subscapularis

The most common surgical exposure used in shoulder arthroplasty is the deltopectoral approach. This approach uses the interval between the deltoid and pectoralis major. In the deeper surgical plane, takedown of the subscapularis tendon is required to gain access to the glenohumeral joint. In anatomic TSA, healing of the subscapularis tendon is essential for success of the procedure, as failure to heal can lead to pain, dysfunction, and instability.[4,5] Many methods of subscapularis takedown have been developed to maximize exposure while minimizing risk of failure after surgery, but the main techniques used today are the subscapularis tenotomy, subscapularis peel, and lesser tuberosity osteotomy (LTO).

Subscapularis tenotomy

The glenohumeral joint was classically accessed via a tenotomy of the subscapularis tendon. In this approach, the subscapularis tendon is transected from proximal to distal, leaving a 1-cm cuff of tendon attached to the lesser tuberosity.[6] The subscapularis tenotomy is an attractive option

for access to the joint, as it is quick and easy to perform, and avoids the risks of nonunion and malunion that are seen with the LTO.

However, there has been concern about tendon-to-tendon suture repair when the tenotomy is used, and its predilection for failure at the suture-tendon junction. In addition, some studies show a high incidence of abnormal subscapularis function after arthroplasty using a tenotomy approach. Miller and colleagues performed a study of patients who received a TSA using a subscapularis tenotomy. On physical examination, their cohort of patients had a 67.5% incidence of abnormal lift-off and a 66.6% incidence of abnormal belly-press. Of the patients with an abnormal lift-off, 92% reported subscapularis dysfunction demonstrated by an inability to tuck in their shirt.[7] Conversely, Caplan and colleagues, in a cohort of 43 TSA patients who underwent a subscapularis tenotomy, showed much better results. Forty-one of 43 patients in their study had a negative lift-off test and all 43 patients had a negative belly-press. They report that relaxing sutures, by way of closing the lateral rotator interval, as well as limiting patients' postoperative external rotation, aid in protecting the subscapularis repair, thereby preventing subscapularis dysfunction.[8]

To avoid some of the setbacks associated with the traditional tenotomy, some variations on the technique have been created. Henderson described an apex-medial V-shaped subscapularis tenotomy. The purpose of the V-shape is to maximize the contact area for tendon to heal, allowing more sutures to be used, which hypothetically leads to a stronger repair. In addition, as the tendon incision is approximately 60° from the line of pull of the muscle, there is decreased chance of suture cut-through compared with repair of a traditional tenotomy.

Subscapularis peel

In the subscapularis peel technique, the tendon is elevated off its insertion onto the lesser tuberosity. The tendon is typically repaired at the end of the case through bone tunnels or using suture anchors. Although there has been concern about tendon healing to bone based on rotator cuff repair literature,[9–12] several biomechanical studies have shown equivalent performance to other subscapularis management techniques.[13,14] An advantage of the peel is the ability to medialize the tendon if necessary.[15]

Lapner and colleagues sought to compare the LTO and peel techniques in a randomized controlled trial. They found no difference in outcome scores or strength at 2 years.[16] The same group compared the peel and tenotomy techniques in another randomized controlled trial. They again found no difference in outcome scores, internal rotation strength, as well as tendon integrity on ultrasound at 2 years.[17] Interestingly, their outcomes for the tenotomy technique were better than were previously reported. This may be due to their repair technique, which used high-tensile strength sutures passed through transosseous tunnels and tied over a miniplate on the greater tuberosity as a reinforcement of the side-to-side repair of the tendon.

Lesser tuberosity osteotomy

The LTO technique was initially proposed as a method to attain more reliable healing via bone-to-bone contact.[18] A 5- to 10-mm lesser tuberosity fragment is created with either an osteotome or saw, and the subscapularis and tuberosity are mobilized as a unit. At the conclusion of the case, the tuberosity is repaired back down in its anatomic position using nonabsorbable sutures through transosseous tunnels (**Fig. 2**). The theoretic advantages of the LTO include the improved healing rates of bone to bone rather than tendon to bone as well as the ability to identify failures more readily on postoperative axillary radiographs with noted displacement of the osteotomy fragment. The downside to the LTO is the possibility of malunion or nonunion of the osteotomy. In a cohort of 189 TSA patients, Levy found an 8.9% rate of displaced tuberosity nonunion. The patients with displaced nonunion had significantly lower functional scores and higher pain scores.[19]

Scalise and colleagues compared patients who underwent shoulder arthroplasty using a tenotomy to those who received an LTO. Although both groups improved substantially from preoperative outcome scores, they found that postoperatively, the LTO group had higher scores with more intact subscapularis tendons on ultrasound. Radiographically, all osteotomies healed in their study.[20] Jandhyala and colleagues similarly found superior TSA patient function after LTO when compared with tenotomy. They created a graded belly-press test to assess the subscapularis postoperatively. They found that the LTO group had significantly better graded belly-press scores, indicating better subscapularis function.[21]

Subscapularis-sparing approaches

Several surgical approaches to the shoulder have been described that avoid taking down the subscapularis. This can be beneficial for the patient's recovery, as the patient does not have to protect a subscapularis repair during early rehabilitation and can begin active motion more quickly. Patient selection is usually reserved for smaller patients and those with less deformity of bony architecture, however, as the exposure can be difficult otherwise.

Lafosse described a superolateral approach to the shoulder for arthroplasty, in which the procedure is performed through the rotator interval. Access to the interval is gained through a deltoid-split but requires subperiosteal elevation of the anterior portion of the deltoid off

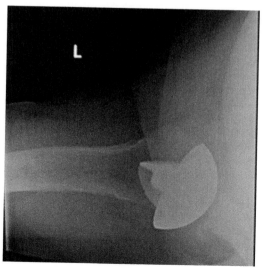

Fig. 2. Axillary radiograph demonstrating a stemless anatomic total shoulder arthroplasty with a well-reduced lesser tuberosity osteotomy.

the acromion. Patients were allowed unrestricted movement with a physical therapist starting on postoperative day 1. The patients in their cohort had good functional outcomes and range of motion scores; however, there were a significant number of patients with nonanatomic neck cuts, residual inferior osteophytes, and undersized humeral head components.[22]

Ross and colleagues described a technique coined the "subscapularis-sparing windowed anterior technique" (SWAT) for TSA. In their technique, a standard deltopectoral incision is made. Rather than releasing the subscapularis, a window inferior to the subscapularis is made to release the inferior capsule and excise any osteophytes, and an anterior window is made through the rotator interval for access to perform the arthroplasty. If there is difficulty with exposure, the standard incision allows for conversion to traditional subscapularis-takedown approaches. In a cohort of 47 patients, they reported that the predicted center of rotation of the native humeral head differed from that of the prosthetic humeral head by only 2.28 mm. In addition, they reported radiographic evidence of successful removal of osteophytes in 75% of cases. They kept their patients in a sling for 2 weeks to allow for soft tissue rest, then encouraged unrestricted motion of the shoulder.[23]

In Reverse Shoulder Arthroplasty
The biomechanics of the shoulder are changed significantly in reverse shoulder arthroplasty (RSA), necessitating a different perspective on the rotator cuff. As opposed to the anatomic shoulder arthroplasty, in which an attempt is made at replicating the native anatomy, the implants in a reverse are semiconstrained and the "ball and socket" are reversed. In addition, the center-of-rotation of the shoulder is shifted medially and inferiorly. This design causes the deltoid to gain a mechanical advantage in terms of elevation, allowing it to effectively move the shoulder and obviating the need for a functioning rotator cuff. For these reasons, the necessity of a subscapularis repair after RSA has come into question.

Proponents of repair the subscapularis in RSA often cite the subscapularis' role as a passive restraint to anterior translation, causing a reduction in the risk of dislocation. Cheung and colleagues retrospectively reviewed a cohort of patients who underwent RSA at their institution. They found a 9.2% rate of postoperative dislocation, and cited male gender, irreparable subscapularis, previous open shoulder surgery, and a

diagnosis of fracture sequelae to be risk factors of instability. They found that an irreparable subscapularis was an independent predictor for instability.[24] Similarly, Edwards and colleagues reviewed a cohort of 138 consecutive RSAs performed by a single surgeon and found that an irreparable subscapularis presented a relative risk of 1.90 for dislocation of the prosthesis.[25]

Those opposed to subscapularis repair state that there is no difference in functional outcomes or complications with no subscapularis repair in modern prostheses. Friedman and associates performed a database study comparing 340 patients who underwent RSA with subscapularis repair to 251 patients who underwent RSA without subscapularis repair. All surgeries were performed using an implant with a lateralized humeral design. They found no difference in complication rate between the repair and no-repair groups. The dislocation rate was 0% in the repair group and 1.2% in the no-repair group, which was not significantly different. They did find that the repair group had better internal rotation, whereas the no-repair group had better abduction and passive external rotation.[26] Similarly, Vourazeris and colleagues reviewed 202 RSA cases performed by one surgeon using an implant with a lateralized humerus. They found no significant difference in outcome scores, range of motion, strength, or complications, including dislocations, between patients who did or did not have a subscapularis repair.[27]

Some have speculated that patients are actually worse off when having the subscapularis repaired in the setting of a lateralized implant. Werner and colleagues reviewed a database of patients who had undergone RSA. They found that patients who had a lateralized implant with subscapularis repair had significantly less improvement than those without a lateralized implant or without subscapularis repair.[28] The reason is thought to be due to the altered vector of pull of the subscapularis muscle. During an RSA, the new position of the humerus causes the subscapularis to function more as an adductor. In turn, the subscapularis becomes antagonistic to the deltoid muscle. This can be accentuated in a lateralized implant, where the subscapularis can experience supraphysiologic tension beyond its anatomic length. In addition, the extra tension works counter to the posterior cuff muscles, causing increased energy requirements for external rotation, particularly in cases with preexisting external rotation weakness.[29,30] These issues can result in the appearance of a functional "hornblower's" sign.

Reverse Shoulder Arthroplasty with Deficient Posterior Cuff

Patients with rotator cuff arthropathy due to posterosuperior rotator cuff tears are routinely treated with RSA. Deficiency of the posterior cuff, particularly with involvement of the teres minor, can present a difficult problem. With Grammont-style implants, these patients have been reported to have trouble with activities of daily living and lower functional outcome scores.[31,32] There are multiple techniques available to address this issue.

Tendon transfer has traditionally been the mainstay of treatment of RSA patients who lack external rotation. The modified L'Episcopo procedure, in which the latissimus dorsi and teres major are transferred as a unit to the lateral humerus, has been reported extensively with good functional results (Fig. 3).[33–35] A problem that can arise with the modified L'Episcopo is that after transfer of the teres major and latissimus dorsi, the pectoralis major is potentially the only internal rotator left attached, assuming the subscapularis is irreparable or not repaired. To combat this issue, an isolated latissimus dorsi transfer can be performed to reestablish external rotation. In this procedure, the latissimus is released in isolation, transferred through a split in the teres major, and reattached to the lateral humerus. Popescu and colleagues

published on a series of patients who underwent RSA with concomitant latissimus dorsi transfer. Their patients reported good outcome scores and ability to perform ADLs.[36] With either of these procedures, the surgeon must be cognizant of the proximity of neurovascular structures. The radial nerve lies on the anterior aspect of the latissimus and teres major tendons and is less than 3 cm away from the medial border of the humerus. The axillary nerve is about 1.4 cm proximal to the superior edge of the teres major.[37]

More recently, the use of lateralized implants has been proposed to treat patients deficient in external rotation. Lateralized implants are thought to better tension the remaining rotator cuff, and to recruit more posterior deltoid fibers to act as external rotators.[38–40] Kwapisz and colleagues reviewed a group of patients who underwent RSA with lateralized prostheses. When comparing patients with Fuchs stage III fatty degeneration of the teres minor and infraspinatus to patients with Fuchs stage II or lower, there was no significant difference in outcome scores or range of motion.[41] Similarly, Berglund and colleagues reviewed patients who underwent RSA with a lateralized implant, had preexisting combined loss of active elevation and external rotation (CLEER), and had not received a tendon transfer. The group found that patients with

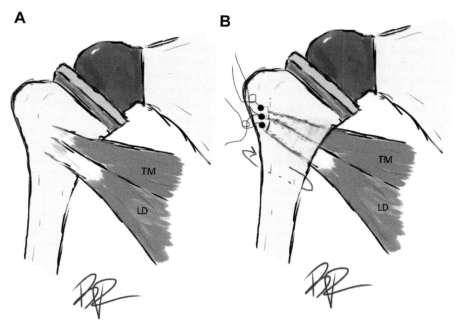

A **B**

Fig. 3. (*A*) Illustration of the insertion sites of the teres major (TM) and latissimus dorsi (LD). (*B*) Illustration of the modified L'Episcopo procedure, in which the LD and TM are transferred around the posterior humerus and reattached on the lateral humerus to restore active external rotation.

CLEER were able to regain a significant amount of external rotation using only a lateralized RSA implant.[42]

LONG HEAD BICEPS TENDON

The tendon of the long head of the biceps (LHB) brachii is encountered during the approach to the glenohumeral joint in its groove between the greater and lesser tuberosities. In shoulder arthroplasty, the tendon is routinely released before taking down the subscapularis tendon and entering the joint. This not only improves visualization of the glenoid for the surgeon[43] but also removes a source of potential shoulder pain in TSA patients.[44,45]

The tendon of the LHB enters the glenohumeral joint through the rotator interval. Because of the intraarticular nature of the tendon, the LHB is commonly affected in the degenerative joint disease process simultaneously. At the microscopic level, the intraarticular portion of the tendon tends to show more degenerative changes than the extraarticular portion.[46] This degeneration leads to the LHB having a role as a potential pain generator, which further supports its removal.

When taking down the LHB tendon, the surgeon can either choose to perform a tenodesis or a tenotomy. The tenodesis is commonly performed by suturing the residual biceps tendon to the tendon of the pectoralis major.

Godeneche and colleagues retrospectively reviewed 268 anatomic arthroplasties performed at their institution. They found that patients who received an LHB tenodesis had significantly better pain scores as well as adjusted Constant scores than patients in whom the biceps was preserved.[47] Fama and his group performed a multicenter study of patients who underwent shoulder arthroplasty using the same prosthesis. They compared outcomes for patients who received an LH7B tenodesis to those who did not. The tenodesis patients had better Constant scores, as well as subjective outcomes of surgery.[48] Simmen also compared arthroplasty patients who received a tenodesis to those who did not in a prospective study. They found that tenodesis patients were more likely to have a successful outcome as defined by a Constant score $\geq$ 80.[49]

A tenotomy is another option for management of the LHB tendon. This procedure still offers the same benefits as the tenodesis at the level of the shoulder; however, the tenotomy can potentially cause increased rates of arm cramping and cosmetic deformity.[50–52] To our knowledge, there are no studies comparing LHB tenotomy and tenodesis in shoulder arthroplasty patients.

GLENOHUMERAL CAPSULE

After release of the subscapularis, management of the capsule becomes important for visualization, as well as soft tissue balancing. The capsule in the arthritic shoulder is often tight and contracted. To begin capsular releases, the anterior capsule is first either excised or released. This helps with exposure of the glenoid, as well as mobilization of the subscapularis. This is followed by excision of the glenoid labrum, and release of the inferior capsule. These releases will allow for subscapularis mobilization, glenoid exposure, and access for appropriate glenoid reaming.[43,53,54] Care is to be taken when releasing the inferior capsule, as the axillary nerve is approximately 1 cm from the inferior glenoid rim and has been reported to be as close as 5.6 mm.[55,56] In RSA, releasing the inferior capsule is also extremely important for stability. If left intact, the humeral component can lever off the tight capsule when the arm is in adduction, providing a mechanism for dislocation.[57,58] This is of particular concern when the goal of glenosphere placement is often as low as possible on the glenoid.

After placement of an anatomic arthroplasty, proper soft tissue tension is commonly assessed by translating the humeral head anteriorly and posteriorly, with 50% translation in both directions routinely used as the goal, although there is limited evidence to support this.[53] As glenohumeral arthritis progresses, the anterior soft tissue structures contract, causing posterior subluxation of the humeral head. As contact pressure increases in the posterior glenohumeral joint, the posterior glenoid becomes worn and the posterior soft tissue structures become stretched.[59–61] The posterior glenoid wear and stretched posterior capsule can cause problems with soft tissue balance with continued posterior subluxation of the humeral head after the procedure.

There have been multiple procedures described to address this problem on the bony glenoid side including corrective high-side reaming, structural bone grafting, augmented glenoid components, and RSA. On the soft-tissue side, plication of the posterior capsule has been described as a technique to address residual laxity.[62] Walch and colleagues published on the results of anatomic TSA in patients with a biconcave glenoid. In their cohort of 92 patients, 9 underwent plication of the posterior capsule.

These patients were found to have decreased forward elevation and performed worse on the mobility aspect of the Constant score.[63] Alentorn-Geli showed that although plication can correct intraoperative posterior instability, there is a high incidence of complications, and the posterior instability can recur in approximately one-third of patients.[64,65] Overall, expectations for success of posterior capsular plication should be limited.

SUMMARY

The success of TSA is strongly dependent on the handling, release, and repair of the surrounding soft tissues. Although proper bony cuts and implant placement can afford the patient good functional outcomes, there are significant limitations when soft tissue repair and balance are not accounted for during shoulder arthroplasty. Ensuring that the patient has a functional rotator cuff before surgery is key in determining whether he or she will benefit more from an anatomic or RSA. And as the takedown of the subscapularis remains the most common approach to shoulder arthroplasty, its proper repair is essential for a good functional outcome and implant longevity in anatomic TSA. Regardless of which technique for subscapularis takedown is used, it is important that the treating surgeon feels comfortable in reproducing good results. In addition, careful release of capsular soft tissue and intraoperative assessment of balance and stability are paramount to good results.

CLINICS CARE POINTS

- Subscapularis repair in anatomic total shoulder arthroplasty is paramount to successful functional outcomes.
- Various options for subscapularis takedown exist and all are successful with proper repair.
- Proper capsular release should not be overlooked as it both improves visualization during surgery and improves patient range of motion outcomes post-operatively.

DISCLOSURE

B.A. Romero: Nothing to disclose. J.G. Horneff: Miami Device Solutions: paid consultant; Tigon Medical: unpaid consultant; OREF: research support; AAOS/ASES: board or committee member.

REFERENCES

1. Zmistowski B, Padegimas EM, Howley M, et al. Trends and variability in the use of total shoulder arthroplasty for medicare patients. J Am Acad Orthop Surg 2018;26(4):133–41.
2. Burkhart SS. Reconciling the paradox of rotator cuff repair versus debridement: a unified biomechanical rationale for the treatment of rotator cuff tears. Arthroscopy 1994;10(1):4–19.
3. Franklin JL, Barrett WP, Jackins SE, et al. Glenoid loosening in total shoulder arthroplasty: association with rotator cuff deficiency. J Arthroplasty 1988;3(1):39–46.
4. Moeckel BH, Altchek DW, Warren RF, et al. Instability of the shoulder after arthroplasty. J Bone Joint Surg 1993;75-A(4):492–7.
5. Baumgarten KM, Osborn R, Schweinle WE, et al. The influence of anatomic total shoulder arthroplasty using a subscapularis tenotomy on shoulder strength. J Shoulder Elbow Surg 2018;27(1):82–9.
6. Rowe CR, Patel D, Southmayd WW. The bankart procedure: a long-term end-result study. J Bone Joint Surg 1978;60(1):1–16.
7. Miller SL, Hazrati Y, Klepps S, et al. Loss of subscapularis function after total shoulder replacement: a seldom recognized problem. J Shoulder Elbow Surg 2003;12(1):29–34.
8. Caplan JL, Whitfield B, Neviaser RJ. Subscapularis function after primary tendon to tendon repair in patients after replacement arthroplasty of the shoulder. J Shoulder Elbow Surg 2009;18(2):193–6.
9. Kwon J, Kim SH, Lee YH, et al. The rotator cuff healing index: a new scoring system to predict rotator cuff healing after surgical repair. Am J Sports Med 2019;47(1):173–80.
10. McElvany MD, McGoldrick E, Gee AO, et al. Rotator cuff repair: published evidence on factors associated with repair integrity and clinical outcome. Am J Sports Med 2015;43(2):491–500.
11. Le BTN, Wu XL, Lam PH, et al. Factors predicting rotator cuff retears: an analysis of 1000 consecutive rotator cuff repairs. Am J Sports Med 2014;42(5):1134–42.
12. Chung SW, Oh JH, Gong HS, et al. Factors affecting rotator cuff healing after arthroscopic repair: osteoporosis as one of the independent risk factors. Am J Sports Med 2011;39(10):2099–107.
13. van Thiel GS, Wang VM, Wang FC, et al. Biomechanical similarities among subscapularis repairs after shoulder arthroplasty. J Shoulder Elbow Surg 2010;19(5):657–63.
14. Virk MS, Aiyash SS, Frank RM, et al. Biomechanical comparison of subscapularis peel and lesser tuberosity osteotomy for double-row subscapularis repair technique in a cadaveric arthroplasty model. J Orthop Surg Res 2019;14(1).

15. Shields E, Ho A, Wiater JM. Management of the subscapularis tendon during total shoulder arthroplasty. J Shoulder Elbow Surg 2017;26(4):723–31.

16. Lapner PLC, Sabri E, Rakhra K, et al. Comparison of lesser tuberosity osteotomy to subscapularis peel in shoulder arthroplasty: a randomized controlled trial. J Bone Joint Surg Am 2012;94(24):2239–46.

17. Lapner P, Pollock JW, Zhang T, et al. A randomized controlled trial comparing subscapularis tenotomy with peel in anatomic shoulder arthroplasty. J Shoulder Elbow Surg 2020;29(2):225–34.

18. Gerber C, Yian EH, Pfirrmann CAW, et al. Subscapularis muscle function and structure after total shoulder replacement with lesser tuberosity osteotomy and repair. J Bone Joint Surg Am 2005;87(8): 1739–45. Available at. www.aaos.org.

19. Levy JC, DeVito P, Berglund D, et al. Lesser tuberosity osteotomy in total shoulder arthroplasty: impact of radiographic healing on outcomes. J Shoulder Elbow Surg 2019;28(6):1082–90.

20. Scalise JJ, Ciccone J, Iannotti JP. Clinical, radiographic, and ultrasonographic comparison of subscapularis tenotomy and lesser tuberosity osteotomy for total shoulder arthroplasty. J Bone Joint Surg Am 2010;92(7):1627–34.

21. Jandhyala S, Unnithan A, Hughes S, et al. Subscapularis tenotomy versus lesser tuberosity osteotomy during total shoulder replacement: a comparison of patient outcomes. J Shoulder Elbow Surg 2011;20(7):1102–7.

22. Lafosse L, Schnaser E, Haag M, et al. Primary total shoulder arthroplasty performed entirely thru the rotator interval: technique and minimum two-year outcomes. J Shoulder Elbow Surg 2009;18(6): 864–73.

23. Ross JP, Lee A, Neeley R, et al. The subscapularis-sparing windowed anterior technique for total shoulder arthroplasty. J Shoulder Elbow Surg 2021;30(7):S89–99.

24. Cheung Ev, Sarkissian EJ, Sox-Harris A, et al. Instability after reverse total shoulder arthroplasty. J Shoulder Elbow Surg 2018;27(11):1946–52.

25. Edwards TB, Williams MD, Labriola JE, et al. Subscapularis insufficiency and the risk of shoulder dislocation after reverse shoulder arthroplasty. J Shoulder Elbow Surg 2009;18(6):892–6.

26. Friedman RJ, Flurin PH, Wright TW, et al. Comparison of reverse total shoulder arthroplasty outcomes with and without subscapularis repair. J Shoulder Elbow Surg 2017;26(4):662–8.

27. Vourazeris JD, Wright TW, Struk AM, et al. Primary reverse total shoulder arthroplasty outcomes in patients with subscapularis repair versus tenotomy. J Shoulder Elbow Surg 2017;26(3):450–7.

28. Werner BC, Wong AC, Mahony GT, et al. Clinical outcomes after reverse shoulder arthroplasty with and without subscapularis repair: the importance of considering glenosphere lateralization. J Am Acad Orthop Surg 2018;26(5):e114–9.

29. Giles JW, Langohr GDG, Johnson JA, et al. The rotator cuff muscles are antagonists after reverse total shoulder arthroplasty. J Shoulder Elbow Surg 2016;25(10):1592–600.

30. Eno JJT, Kontaxis A, Novoa-Boldo A, et al. The biomechanics of subscapularis repair in reverse shoulder arthroplasty: The effect of lateralization and insertion site. J Orthop Res 2020;38(4):888–94.

31. Sirveaux F, Favard L, Oudet D, et al. Grammont inverted total shoulder arthroplasty in the treatment of glenohumeral osteoarthritis with massive rupture of the cuff: Results of a multicentre study of 80 shoulders. J Bone Joint Surg Br 2004;86: 388–95.

32. Boileau P, Watkinson D, Hatzidakis AM, et al. Neer award 2005: the grammont reverse shoulder prosthesis: results in cuff tear arthritis, fracture sequelae, and revision arthroplasty. J Shoulder Elbow Surg 2006;15(5):527–40.

33. Shi LL, Cahill KE, Ek ET, et al. Latissimus dorsi and teres major transfer with reverse shoulder arthroplasty restores active motion and reduces pain for posterosuperior cuff dysfunction. Clin Orthop Relat Res 2015;473(10):3212–7.

34. Boileau P, Rumian AP, Zumstein MA. Reversed shoulder arthroplasty with modified L'Episcopo for combined loss of active elevation and external rotation. J Shoulder Elbow Surg 2010;19(2 Suppl): 20–30.

35. Boileau P, Chuinard C, Roussanne Y, et al. Modified latissimus dorsi and teres major transfer through a single delto-pectoral approach for external rotation deficit of the shoulder: As an isolated procedure or with a reverse arthroplasty. J Shoulder Elbow Surg 2007;16(6):671–82.

36. Popescu IA, Bihel T, Henderson D, et al. Functional improvements in active elevation, external rotation, and internal rotation after reverse total shoulder arthroplasty with isolated latissimus dorsi transfer: surgical technique and midterm follow-up. J Shoulder Elbow Surg 2019;28(12):2356–63.

37. Pearle AD, Kelly BT, Voos JE, et al. Surgical technique and anatomic study of latissimus dorsi and teres major transfers. J Bone Joint Surg Am 2006; 88(7):1524–31.

38. Valenti P, Sauzières P, Katz D, et al. Do less medialized reverse shoulder prostheses increase motion and reduce notching? Clin Orthop Relat Res 2011; 469(9):2550–7.

39. Frankle M, Siegal S, Pupello D, et al. The reverse shoulder prosthesis for glenohumeral arthritis associated with severe rotator cuff deficiency: a minimum two-year follow-up study of sixty patients. J Bone Joint Surg Am 2005;87(8):1697–705. Available at. www.jbjs.org.

40. Greiner S, Schmidt C, Herrmann S, et al. Clinical performance of lateralized versus non-lateralized reverse shoulder arthroplasty: a prospective randomized study. J Shoulder Elbow Surg 2015;24(9):1397–404.

41. Kwapisz A, Rogers JP, Thigpen CA, et al. Infraspinatus or teres minor fatty infiltration does not influence patient outcomes after reverse shoulder arthroplasty with a lateralized glenoid. JSES Int 2021;5(1):109–13.

42. Berglund DD, Rosas S, Triplet JJ, et al. Restoration of external rotation following reverse shoulder arthroplasty without latissimus dorsi transfer. JB JS Open Access 2018;3(2):1–8.

43. Lovse LJ, Culliton K, Pollock JW, et al. Glenoid exposure in shoulder arthroplasty: the role of soft tissue releases. JSES Int 2020;4(2):377–81.

44. Hersch JC, Dines DM. Arthroscopy for failed shoulder arthroplasty. Arthroscopy 2000;16(6):606–12.

45. Tuckman Dv, Dines DM. Long head of the biceps pathology as a cause of anterior shoulder pain after shoulder arthroplasty. J Shoulder Elbow Surg 2006; 15(4):415–8.

46. Mazzocca AD, McCarthy MBR, Ledgard FA, et al. Histomorphologic changes of the long head of the biceps tendon in common shoulder pathologies. Arthroscopy 2013;29(6):972–81.

47. Godenèche A, Boileau P, Favard L, et al. Prosthetic replacement in the treatment of osteoarthritis of the shoulder: early results of 208 cases. J Shoulder Elbow Surg 2002;11(1):11–8.

48. Fama G, Edwards B, Boulahia A, et al. The role of concomitant biceps tenodesis in shoulder arthroplasty for primary osteoarthritis: results of a multicentric study. Orthopedics 2004;27(4):401–5.

49. Simmen BR, Bachmann LM, Drerup S, et al. Usefulness of concomitant biceps tenodesis in total shoulder arthroplasty: a prospective cohort study. J Shoulder Elbow Surg 2008;17(6):921–4.

50. Virk MS, Nicholson GP. Complications of proximal biceps tenotomy and tenodesis. Clin Sports Med 2016;35(1):181–8.

51. MacDonald P, Verhulst F, McRae S, et al. Biceps tenodesis versus tenotomy in the treatment of lesions of the long head of the biceps tendon in patients undergoing arthroscopic shoulder surgery: a prospective double-blinded randomized controlled trial. Am J Sports Med 2020;48(6):1439–49.

52. Hsu AR, Ghodadra NS, Provencher CMT, et al. Biceps tenotomy versus tenodesis: a review of clinical outcomes and biomechanical results. J Shoulder Elbow Surg 2011;20(2):326–32.

53. Ibarra C, Craig E v. Soft-tissue balancing in total shoulder arthroplasty. Orthop Clin North Am 1998;29(3):415–22.

54. Nové-Josserand L, Clavert P. Glenoid exposure in total shoulder arthroplasty. Orthop Traumatol-Sur Res 2018;104(1):S129–35.

55. Makki D, Selmi H, Syed S, et al. How close is the axillary nerve to the inferior glenoid? a magnetic resonance study of normal and arthritic shoulders. Ann R Coll Surg Engl 2020;102(6):408–11.

56. Hachadorian ME, Mitchell BC, Siow MY, et al. Identifying the axillary nerve during shoulder surgery: an anatomic study using advanced imaging. JSES Int 2020;4(4):987–91.

57. Chalmers PN, Rahman Z, Romeo AA, et al. Early dislocation after reverse total shoulder arthroplasty. J Shoulder Elbow Surg 2014;23(5):737–44.

58. Cheung E, Willis M, Walker M, et al. Complications in reverse total shoulder arthroplasty. J Am Acad Orthop Surg 2011;19(7):439–49.

59. Neer CS. Replacement arthroplasty for glenohumeral osteoarthritis. J Bone Joint Surg Am 1974;56(1):1–13.

60. Neer CS, Watson KC, Stantont FJ. Recent experience in total shoulder replacement. J Bone Joint Surg Am 1982;64(3):319–37.

61. Walch G, Badet R, Boulahia A, et al. Morphologic study of the glenoid in primary glenohumeral osteoarthritis. J Arthroplasty 1999;14(6):756–60.

62. Namba RS, Thornhill TS. Posterior capsulorrhaphy in total shoulder arthroplasty: a case report. Clin Orthop Relat Res 1995;313:135–9.

63. Walch G, Moraga C, Young A, et al. Results of anatomic nonconstrained prosthesis in primary osteoarthritis with biconcave glenoid. J Shoulder Elbow Surg 2012;21(11):1526–33.

64. Alentorn-Geli E, Wanderman NR, Assenmacher AT, et al. Anatomic total shoulder arthroplasty with posterior capsular plication versus reverse shoulder arthroplasty in patients with biconcave glenoids: a matched cohort study. J Orthop Surg 2018;26(2).

65. Alentorn-Geli E, Assenmacher AT, Sperling JW, et al. Plication of the posterior capsule for intraoperative posterior instability during anatomic total shoulder arthroplasty. J Shoulder Elbow Surg 2017;26(6):982–9.

Foot and Ankle

Plantar Plate Repair for Metatarsophalangeal Joint Instability of the Lesser Toes

James R. Jastifer, MD[a,b,*]

KEYWORDS

- Crossover toe • MTP instability • Plantar plate tear • Plantar plate repair

---

KEY POINTS

- Plantar plate tears are recognized as a cause of metatarsalgia
- Clinical staging and anatomic grading criteria have been published to guide the surgeons on the treatment of MTP instability
- Direct surgical repair of the plantar plate is an option in cases refractory to conservative treatment.

NATURE OF THE PROBLEM

Although a plantar plate tear is a common cause of metatarsalgia, there are many other possible causes of metatarsophalangeal (MTP) joint pain and pathology that may be encountered by the practicing orthopedic surgeon[1–3] (**Box 1**). The link between deformity and pathology as it relates to a plantar plate tear stems from the 1987 publication by Coughlin,[4] who coined the term "second crossover toe" to characterize the clinical deformity of the second toe extending at the MTP joint, and crossing over the great toe medially. Today, this is recognized as a late finding in the clinical course. Early in the disease process, the clinical presentation of pain at the base of the proximal phalanx and associated swelling at the MTP joint may be noted. Subtle deviation of the toe at the level of the MTP joint, either clinically or radiographically, may be appreciated as well. It can be also noted that the second toe is almost exclusively involved but other toes have been associated with this deformity.[1,5–9] Because of the almost exclusive involvement of the second toe, the term "second crossover toe" as described by Coughlin has been widely adapted when referring to this

pathologic condition. Although the cause of MTP instability is ultimately unknown, it is thought to be multifactorial, and may have an acute or insidious clinical course. These challenges have spurred researchers in recent years to develop new clinical and surgical grading systems to further define the pathologic condition.[9–12] Historically, surgical treatment included some combination of MTP soft tissue release, flexor to extensor tendon transfer, extensor tendon lengthening, Weil osteotomy, and Kirschner wire fixation. As described in this review, more recently, direct plantar plate repair is a surgical treatment option.

ANATOMY OF THE PLANTAR PLATE

The plantar plate is thought to be an important contributor to MTP instability.[13] The plantar plate, a flexible but inelastic ligament, measures an average of 19 mm in length and 2 mm in thickness.[14,15] The plantar plate originates on the plantar metatarsal head just proximal to the articular margin and inserts distally on the plantar base of the proximal phalanx.[2,16,17] This insertion is immediately adjacent to the articular surface and is where distal plantar plate tears can be

---

[a] Ascension Borgess Orthopedics, 2490 South 11th Street, Kalamazoo, MI, USA; [b] Western Michigan University Homer Stryker M.D. School of Medicine, Kalamazoo, MI, USA
* Corresponding author.
E-mail address: jrjast@gmail.com

Orthop Clin N Am 53 (2022) 349–359
https://doi.org/10.1016/j.ocl.2022.02.002
0030-5898/22/© 2022 Elsevier Inc. All rights reserved.

visualized. The dorsal appearance of the plantar plate is pseudoarticular, because it is intra-articular and contacts the articular surface of the metatarsal head. The ligament, which is made of 75% type 1 collagen with minimal to no elastin, has fibers oriented longitudinally with some inter-woven oblique fibers, which supports the notion that its strength is in resisted longitudinal tension.[14,15] The plantar aspect is centrally grooved to accommodate the flexor tendons, which reside plantar to the plantar plate. This can be a distinguishing characteristic during a plantar approach to the ligament. The function of the plantar plate can be thought of as a combination of resistance to forces during weight-bearing and joint stability. The plantar plate provides cushioning to the MTP joint during weight-bearing and to be the primary restraint against tensile loads in the sagittal plane.[3,7] Because of the central and plantar location, the extension to the collateral ligaments, and thickness, it is thought that the plantar plate itself is a major stabilizing structure of the MTP joint.[3,18,19] This fact has been supported by multiple studies that have shown a link between the integrity of the plantar plate and instability of the MTP joint.[1,10,14,20–22] Insufficiency of the plantar and associated collateral ligament dysfunction may lead to sagittal and transverse plane instability and deformity.[23,24] Studies have shown that the pathology of the plantar plate is typically located at the insertion near the base of the proximal phalanx.[2,10,15,16,18,20,21,25]

The relationship between anatomy and functional MTP stability is complex. Chalayon and colleagues[13] performed a study examining the sagittal plane stability of the MTP joint. The investigators examined the intact MTP joint compared with a plantar plate disruption, and then to a Weil osteotomy as treatment of the plantar plate disruption and a flexor to extensor tendon transfer as a treatment of the plantar plate disruption.[13] It was noted that the plantar plate significantly contributed to the MTP joint

sagittal stability. The Weil osteotomy created further instability and a flexor to extensor tendon transfer increased stability but not to the intact level. Based on these data, it was concluded that direct plantar plate repair is needed to restore the mechanics of the MTP joint.

The function of the plantar plate is to provide passive resistance to dorsiflexion and participate in active resistance through peripheral attachment of the intrinsic muscles of the foot, which helps prevents hyperdorsiflexion. Plantar plate insufficiency allows dorsal subluxation of the proximal phalanx on the metatarsal head. This subluxation of the joint moves the line of action of the interossei muscles dorsal to the axis of rotation of the MTP joint, and thus they act as a dorsiflexor of the MTP joint as opposed to a plantar flexor, which further exacerbates the deformity. The lumbrical also has an important role due to its medial location at the MTP joint; it is tethered by the deep transverse metatarsal ligament and becomes a medially deforming force, thus creating an adduction force vector on the toe and additionally exacerbating the deformity.[10,11,17,26] The collateral ligaments contribute to both transverse and sagittal plane misalignment of the toe.[10,27] Based on these studies, as well as the author's experience, plantar plate insufficiency is a primary pathologic finding that leads to lesser toe instability.[9–11,21,27,28]

DEMOGRAPHICS

Several demographic categories have been associated with MTP instability including a long second metatarsal, acute trauma, chronic inflammatory disease, hallux valgus, hallux varus, hallux rigidus, interdigital neuromas, hammer toe deformities, or pes planovalgus.[5–7,19,21,22,24,29] Fleischer and colleagues[30] noted that disruption of the normal metatarsal parabola, including a long second metatarsal, is a risk factor for developing second MTP joint plantar plate tears. Even still, the cause may be insidious and idiopathic in nature. These pathologic processes, however, likely contribute to an alteration of the biomechanical loading characteristics of the plantar MTP joint. Although traumatic disruption of the plantar plate can lead to instability, more often it is the product of an insidious and idiopathic onset of patient symptoms from attritional changes.[9,22,31,32] This concept of chronic loading conditions as the most common cause is supported by the fact that although MTP instability has been reported in younger male athletes, it is most commonly seen in older females.[1,19] The second toe is most commonly involved,[4] but Nery and colleagues[9] observed in a large series of 55 plantar plate tears (28 patients) that two-thirds of patients had second toe involvement, whereas a third of patients had third or fourth toe involvement.

HISTORY AND PHYSICAL EXAMINATION

The most common presenting symptom of plantar plate tears is pain at the base of the proximal phalanx of the affected toe. Deformity often develops with time and is most commonly a sagittal (dorsiflexion) and coronal (medial deviation) plane deformity because the abnormal mechanics causes tissue attenuation. Other clinical findings that may be associated with MTP joint instability include swelling of the toe, swelling on the plantar aspect of the MTP joint, and intermetatarsal nerve neuritic symptoms.[7,9–11,25]

Observation during standing is important. With standing, and careful comparison with the contralateral foot and unaffected toes, the development of a gap between the adjacent toes or medial deviation of a toe is a frequent finding.[1,5,10,23] Next, dorsiflexion and crossover deformity is seen in later stages, as the deformity progresses.[19] Finally, an associated hammer toe deformity at the proximal interphalangeal joint of the toe can develop and cause dorsal irritation and fixed deformity of the joint.[3,5]

Klein and colleagues[33] performed a study to correlate physical examination findings with intraoperative findings and preoperative clinical findings compared with intraoperative findings. Several associations were noted to be highly sensitive for detecting plantar plate tears including gradual onset of pain (93%), previous first ray surgery (100%, despite an incidence of 18%), pain at the second metatarsal head (98% sensitive), and edema at the second metatarsal head (95.8% sensitive). Acute onset of pain and toe deformity was rare but specific (7% incidence, 100% specificity).[33]

An associated complaint is radiating nerve pain into the affected or adjacent toe, similar to an interdigital neuroma, but may also be a symptom of MTP capsular swelling causing inflammation of the adjacent intermetatarsal space nerve.[34] Coughlin and colleagues[8] noted this has about a 20% incidence. In these cases, performance of a Mulders examination does not typically elicit a "Mulder click," but the symptoms may be similar to a neuroma.[19,34,35] If the diagnosis is still not clinically clear, sequential injections in the adjacent MTP joints and intermetatarsal spaces may help lead to an accurate diagnosis.[5,19,36]

The "drawer test" is a pathognomonic finding associated with MTP joint instability because it is thought to be the most specific finding (80.6% sensitivity, 99.8% specific) (**Fig. 1**).[9,19,33,37] This test is performed by grasping the proximal phalanx of the involved digit and applying a vertical stress in a dorsal direction while stabilizing the metatarsal. This maneuver can reproduce the patient's pain, and the clinician may feel the MTP joint sublux or dislocate dorsally. Another useful test is the "paper pull-out test." Owing to a lack of appropriate intrinsic plantarflexion of the MTP joint (from dorsal displacement of the line of action of the muscle), the plantar flexion strength of the digit may be decreased; this can be quantified by using the "paper pull-out test" (**Fig. 2A,B**).[21] A strip of paper towel is placed under the affected toe tip. The patient attempts to grip the paper, while the examiner pulls the strip. If the paper can be removed without tearing, it is evidence of a plantar plate tear.

Evaluation of the magnitude of deformity and the associated instability on drawer testing allows the clinician to preoperatively stage the condition on a 0 to 4 scale, which can be used in presurgical planning (**Table 1**).

IMAGING STUDIES

Standard 3-view weight-bearing foot radiographs should be obtained to assess for associated deformity and pathology, MTP joint

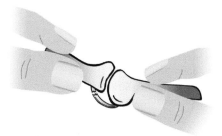 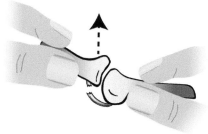

Fig. 1. Drawer test. (*From* Jastifer et al.[59]; with permission.)

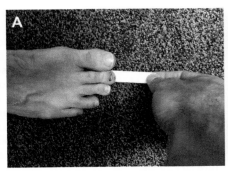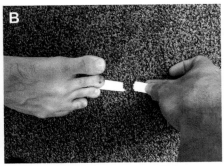

Fig. 2. Photographs of (*A*) before and (*B*) after "paper pull-out test". (*From* Jastifer et al.[59]; with permission.)

congruity, angular deformity of the ray, and arthritic or posttraumatic changes of the foot.[19] Common findings include a disruption in the metatarsal parabola of the foot, with an increase in length of the symptomatic metatarsal, and increase in the 1-2 intermetatarsal angle with associated hallux valgus, and medial deviation of the second toe and splaying of the digits.[30,38]

MRI and ultrasonography have also been described as imaging modalities. Arthrography has been described as useful in determining the presence of plantar plate tears, but it is limited in defining the size or pattern of the tear.[17,28,39] Several investigators have published on evaluating plantar plate tears with MRI. Yao and colleagues[40] were the first to describe this use. Nery and colleagues[9] and Sung and colleagues[41] reported MRI to be both sensitive and specific in determining the presence and extent of plantar plate pathology. In the author's experience, ultrasonography may be considered but the results are highly technician dependent and not reliable. Studies do show, however, that in the hands of a qualified technologist, ultrasonography is more sensitive than MRI (91.5% vs 73.9%), whereas MRI is more specific

(100% vs 25%).[41–43] In the author's experience, the combination of a 3-T MRI with high-resolution cuts through the area of concern and an experienced musculoskeletal radiologist can provide useful diagnostic information, and they no longer use ultrasonography or arthrography to assist in making a diagnosis.

CLASSIFICATION

Classification systems are clinically useful if they guide treatment. Several grading schemes have been developed for use in describing MTP joint instability,[17,26,28,44] but only recently has the plantar plate involvement in lesser MTP joint instability been considered in these classifications.[9–12,14,25,28,45,46]

There are 2 systems published to stage and grade MTP instability of the lesser toes. The first incorporates physical examination findings and many of the principles of previous rating systems[7,9,17,26,28,44] (see **Table 1**). A grading system has also been developed based on anatomic cadaveric dissections of plantar plate dysfunction in cadavers with known MTP instability (**Table 2**). These systems help the clinician

Table 1 Anatomic grading of plantar plate tear	
Grade	**Description**
0	Plantar plate or capsular attenuation, and/or discoloration
I	Transverse distal tear (adjacent to insertion into proximal phalanx [<50%]; medial, lateral, or central area) and/or midsubstance tear (<50%)
II	Transverse distal tear (≥50%); medial, lateral, or central area and/or midsubstance tear (≥50%)
III	Transverse and/or longitudinal extensive tear (may involve collateral ligaments)
IV	Extensive tear with button hole (dislocation)

Table 2
Clinical staging system for second metatarsophalangeal joint

Grade	Alignment	Physical Examination
0	MTP joint; normal alignment. Prodromal phase with pain but no deformity	MTP joint pain, thickening or swelling of the MTP joint, reduced toe purchase, negative drawer
I	Mild malalignment at MTP joint, widening of web space, medial deviation	MTP joint pain, swelling of MTP joint, loss of toe purchase, mild positive drawer (<50% subluxable)
II	Moderate malalignment; medial, lateral, dorsal, or dorsomedial deformity; hyperextension of toe	MTP joint pain, reduced swelling, no toe purchase, moderate positive drawer (≥50% subluxable)
III	Severe malalignment; dorsal or dorsomedial deformity. Second toe can overlap the hallux. May have flexible hammer toe	Joint and toe pain, little swelling, no toe purchase, very positive drawer (dislocatable MTP joint), flexible hammer toe
IV	Very severe deformity: dorsomedial or dorsal dislocation, severe deformity with dislocation, fixed hammer toe	Joint and toe pain, little or no swelling, no toe purchase, dislocated MTP joint, fixed hammer toe

address the dysfunction and quantifying the deformity. Of the tear types, grade 3 tears are the most common, accounting for almost half of all tears (**Figs. 3** and **4A–D**).[9]

CONSERVATIVE TREATMENT

Early diagnosis of plantar plate pathology is difficult because the natural history may be insidious in onset (see **Fig. 4**). It is common for patients to have several years of symptoms and/or deformity before presentation. The hammer toe deformity, a late result of the MTP instability, may be the presenting symptom.[5] Because of

this insidious course, conservative treatment should be exhausted as a first-line treatment (**Fig. 5A–D**). Owing to the anatomic factors driving the malalignment, conservative treatment may reduce painful metatarsalgia, but it is unlikely to alter the deformity.[47] Shoewear modifications such as a roomy toe box can accommodate the deformity and may reduce irritating pressure on the toe. A full-length, full-width, graphite insole with metatarsal pad may also reduce the applied stress across the painful toe during the toe off phase of gait.[6,10,36] If a hammer toe is present, it may be accommodated with traditional toe sleeves or pads. The

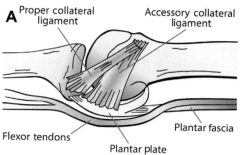
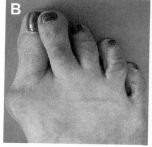
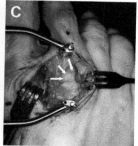

Fig. 3. (*A*) MTP plantar plate anatomy; (*B*) clinical deformity of a crossover second toe associated with hallux valgus; (*C*) grade 3 tear with a tear greater than 50% of the width of the phalanx and proximal extension (*white arrows*). (*From* Jastifer et al.[59]; with permission.)

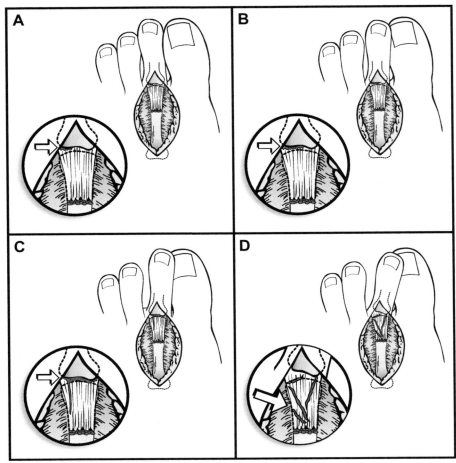

Fig. 4. (*A*) Grade 1, (*B*) grade 2, (*C*) grade 3, and (*D*) grade 4 plantar plate tears. (*From* Jastifer et al.[59]; with permission.)

author has found that taping the affected toe in the early stages of the disease may relieve symptoms associated with activity by providing sagittal plane stability. Taping is generally not successful the worse the deformity gets such as a moderately subluxed or dislocated MTP joint.[5] Coughlin[1,4] reported on a small series of patients with crossover deformity and found that

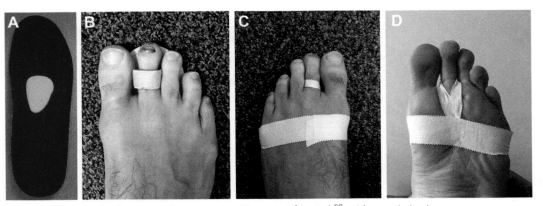

Fig. 5. (*A–D*) Methods of conservative treatment. (*From* Jastifer et al.[59]; with permission.)

although taping of the digit slowed progression of the deformity, patients continued to experience joint pain. Patients should be cautioned that long-term taping may carry the risk of toe ulceration or chronic edema.[6] Selective corticosteroid injections may be used both as a diagnostic and therapeutic option. These injections should be used with caution because they may mask symptoms, contribute to fat pad atrophy, and allow further capsular and plantar plate degeneration.[6,10,36] When a patient determines that conservative treatment has been exhausted and symptoms persist, surgical intervention may be considered.

SURGICAL TREATMENT

Historically, surgical treatment of plantar plate tears included some combination of indirect procedures such as an MTP soft tissue release, flexor to extensor tendon transfer, extensor tendon lengthening, Weil osteotomy, plantar metatarsal condylectomy, and Kirschner wire fixation.[7,17,19,24,44,46,48] Direct repair of the plantar plate has been described both through a plantar approach[21,28,49] and through a straight dorsal approach.[2,9,45] (Fig. 6A, B)

PLANTAR PLATE REPAIR VIA A DORSAL APPROACH (AUTHOR'S PREFERRED METHOD)

1. Positioning: The patient is placed in a supine position on the operating room table. A thigh tourniquet is used to decrease tension on the extrinsic toe tendons.

Regional or general anesthesia is used depending on surgeon preference.[9–11]
2. Incision: A dorsal approach is used via a longitudinal incision centered just lateral to the extensor tendon. The extensor digitorum brevis and longus are retracted medially.
3. Approach and exposure: The medial and lateral collateral ligaments are released from the base of the proximal phalanx of the MTP joint to improve visualization.[50] The medial and lateral collateral ligaments are preserved on the metatarsal head to preserve blood supply. A McGlamry elevator is used to release the proximal aspect of the plantar plate from the first metatarsal, which aids in the proximal proximal translation of the capital fragment.
4. Weil osteotomy: A Weil osteotomy is performed in most cases, although it is not always necessary, using a sagittal saw. The metatarsal head is translated proximally and temporarily fixed with a Kirschner wire. A second Kirschner wire is placed in the proximal phalanx and distraction is applied to the wires across the joint.
5. Visualization: The plantar plate tear is evaluated and graded. If repair is indicated, the remainder of the distal aspect of the plantar plate is released from the proximal phalanx and the plantar aspect of the proximal phalanx is debrided to healthy tissue to improve healing potential.
6. Suture placement: A horizontal mattress suture is placed in the distal stump via a

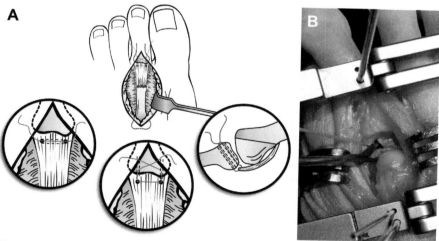

Fig. 6. (*A*) Diagram of dorsal approach for plantar plate repair; (*B*) typical exposure and use of suture passer, note the flexor tendon deep to the plantar plate. (*From* Jastifer et al.[59]; with permission.)

small curved needle or commercially available procedure-specific device. A horizontal mattress is thought to be the strongest suture configuration.[51]

7. Suture passage: Two oblique vertical drill holes (using a 1.5-mm K-wire or 1.6-mm drill) are made on the dorsal medial and dorsal lateral base of the proximal phalanx from dorsal to plantar. The ends of the sutures are then passed from plantar to dorsal with a suture passer and tied over the proximal phalanx bone bridge. This is often the most difficult portion of the procedure. The sutures are tied with the toe in slight (about 20°) plantarflexion.

8. Weil fixation: The Weil osteotomy is fixed with 2 small compression screws, typically with slight shortening. This step is typically performed after suture passage but before tying the suture over the phalanx.

9. Ligament balancing: Coronal plane alignment is assessed, and the lateral capsule is usually tightened if medial deviation of the toe is present. In the rare case that soft tissue balancing alone is not possible, an extensor digitorum brevis transfer to the capsule or temporary Kirschner wire fixation may be considered.

10. Closure: The wound is copiously irrigated and closed with 3-0 Monocryl suture, and a postoperative compressive dressing is applied with the toe held in slight plantarflexion.

11. Postoperative care: Postoperatively, immediate heel weight-bearing in a postoperative shoe is allowed. The patient can transition to commercially available shoes when swelling allows. Flexion and extension passive and active range-of-motion exercises are commenced after surgery to rehabilitate the intrinsic and extrinsic flexors and extensors of the lesser toes.

OUTCOMES

Before the advent of direct plantar plate repair, surgical treatment was limited to indirect methods. The most frequently described techniques included an MTP joint synovectomy,[23] capsular soft tissue release with reefing,[1,4,6,19,31,44,48] extensor and flexor tendon transfers,[1,4,8,17,19,21,26,44,48] phalangeal and metatarsal osteotomies,[7,17,26] and digit amputation.[52] These methods ultimately have frustrated patients and surgeons likely to some degree because they do not address the principal cause of MTP instability, the plantar plate.[4,6,7,9–11,17,26,27,53] The evolution of a dorsal approach to the plantar plate began from an exposure perspective. Cooper and Coughlin,[2] in a cadaveric study, showed that adequate exposure of a lesser MTP joint could be achieved using a dorsal approach and a Weil osteotomy. Jastifer and Coughlin[50] showed that the Weil osteotomy is often not even necessary.

Surgical techniques have evolved to achieve direct repair of plantar plate tears.[9,10,15,21,28,45] Gregg and colleagues[45] published the earliest series, a retrospective series of 35 dorsal plantar plate repairs with Weil osteotomies and noted a 74% patient satisfaction rate. Ford and colleagues[46] published a comparative study including a primary plantar plate repair, a flexor tendon transfer (FTT), and a combined FTT and plantar plate repair. The investigators concluded that a primary plantar plate repair was a viable alternative to FTT in stabilizing the lesser MTP joint. Although the most direct way to access the plantar plate would be from a plantar approach, concern exists over a painful plantar scar. Despite this, a plantar approach has been reported to achieve satisfactory results.[21,28,54] Most recently, Prissel and colleagues[54] published a series of 144 plantar plate repairs through a plantar approach and noted a 4.2% rate of wound complications; only 55.3% of patients reported that they would have the procedure again, and 31.6% of patients reported pain attributed to the plantar scar. The limitation of the plantar approach is the lack of exposure of the MTP joint, and this is important if dorsal release or osteotomies are being considered.

In the largest study to date on dorsal repairs, Flint and colleagues[55] reported on the results of 138 dorsal plantar plate repairs in 97 feet and in 91 patients. The investigators found that 80.4% of patients reported "good" to "excellent" satisfaction scores at 12 months of follow-up. The mean visual analog scale (VAS) pain score improved from 5.4 to 1.5/10, and American Orthopaedic Foot and Ankle Society (AOFAS) scores increased from 49 to 81 points. The investigators note that there was a significant loss of both active and passive range of motion after repair but only 6 had a positive result of drawer examination postoperatively. In another important study, Nery and colleagues[56] report on 100 plantar plate tears treated with thermal shrinkage (grade 0 and grade 1), or plantar plate repair (grade 2 and grade 3), or flexor to extensor tendon transfer (grade 4). Of the 48 repairs treated with plantar plate repair, VAS scores improved from 7.8 to 0.7/10 in the grade 2 tears and from 8 to 1.2/10 in the grade 3 tears.[56] The investigators noted that grade 4 tears had less improvement in pain and only a fair AOFAS average score (72 points) In these studies, grade 4 tears were treated with flexor to extensor tendon transfers, whereas Sung[57] reported a method of reconstruction of the plantar plate using a suture tape and 2 interference screws. As an alternative to a flexor to extensor tendon transfer, the author has performed a flexor tendon tenodesis to the base of the proximal phalanx, which can be performed through the same incision as a dorsal approach; however, no clinical studies have been performed. Cook[58] reported on a retrospective cohort of 50 patients treated with a dorsal anatomic plantar plate repair and noted that 92% demonstrated improved digital stability and 90% had improved radiographic alignment. In another smaller study, Nery and colleagues[9] reported on 22 patients with 40 plantar plate repairs using a dorsal approach and observed substantial relief of pain, correction of deformity, improved MTP joint stability, and an improvement in the mean AOFAS score from 52 to 92 points.

SUMMARY

Plantar plate tears are thought to be the contributing pathology associated with lesser toe MTP instability. Conservative treatment remains the first-line treatment of this pathologic condition. The evolution of surgical treatment to direct surgical repair, although still without long-term data, is thought to be a viable treatment option. Early studies have helped develop a staging system based on the clinical examination, and grading of the tear based on surgical findings. Early surgical outcome studies suggest improved pain scores and relatively high patient satisfaction.

CLINICS CARE POINTS

- Plantar plate tears are a known cause of MTP instability
- Diagnosis of plantar plate tears can reliably be made based on physical examination findings as well as imaging (radiographs, MRI)
- Conservative treatment including shoewear modifications, inserts, and toe taping remains the first-line treatment of plantar plate tears.
- The largest study to date on dorsal repairs reports 80.4% "good" to "excellent" satisfaction scores at 12 months of follow up.[55]

DISCLOSURE

The author has nothing to disclose.

REFERENCES

1. Coughlin MJ. Second metatarsophalangeal joint instability in the athlete. Foot Ankle 1993;14(6):309–19.
2. Cooper MT, Coughlin MJ. Sequential dissection for exposure of the second metatarsophalangeal joint. Foot Ankle Int 2011;32(3):294–9.
3. DuVries HL. Dislocation of the toe. JAMA 1956;160:728.
4. Coughlin MJ. Crossover second toe deformity. Foot Ankle 1987;8(1):29–39.
5. Coughlin MJ. When to suspect crossover second toe deformity. J Musculoskelet Med 1987;39–48.
6. Coughlin MJ. Subluxation and dislocation of the second metatarsophalangeal joint. Orthop Clin North Am 1989;20(4):535–51.
7. Coughlin MJ. Lesser toe deformities. In: Coughlin MJ, Mann CL, Saltzman CL, editors. Surg Foot Ankle, vol. 1, 8th edition. Philadelphia (PA): Mosby Elsevier Inc.; 2007. p. 363–464.
8. Coughlin MJ, Schenck RC Jr, Shurnas PS, et al. Concurrent interdigital neuroma and MTP joint instability: long-term results of treatment. Foot Ankle Int 2002;23(11):1018–25.
9. Nery C, Coughlin MJ, Baumfeld D, et al. Lesser metatarsophalangeal joint instability: prospective evaluation and repair of plantar plate and capsular insufficiency. Foot Ankle Int 2012;33(4):301–11.
10. Coughlin MJ, Baumfeld DS, Nery C. Second MTP joint instability: grading of the deformity and description of surgical repair of capsular insufficiency. Physician Sportsmed 2011;39(3):132–41.
11. Coughlin MJ, Schutt SA, Hirose CB, et al. Metatarsophalangeal joint pathology in crossover second toe deformity: a cadaveric study. Foot Ankle Int 2012;33(2):133–40.
12. Weil L Jr, Sung W, Weil LS, et al. Anatomic plantar plate repair using the Weil metatarsal osteotomy approach. Foot Ankle Spec 2011;4(3):145–50.
13. Chalayon O, Chertman C, Guss AD, et al. Role of plantar plate and surgical reconstruction techniques on static stability of lesser metatarsophalangeal joints: a biomechanical study. Foot Ankle Int 2013;34(10):1436–42.
14. Deland JT, Lee KT, Sobel M, et al. Anatomy of the plantar plate and its attachments in the lesser metatarsal phalangeal joint. Foot Ankle Int 1995;16(8):480–6.
15. Johnston RB 3rd, Smith J, Daniels T. The plantar plate of the lesser toes: an anatomical study in human cadavers. Foot Ankle Int 1994;15(5):276–82.

16. Gregg J, Marks P, Silberstein M, et al. Histologic anatomy of the lesser metatarsophalangeal joint plantar plate. Surg Radiol Anat 2007;29(2):141–7.

17. Mendicino RW, Statler TK, Saltrick KR, et al. Predislocation syndrome: a review and retrospective analysis of eight patients. J foot Ankle Surg 2001;40(4): 214–24.

18. Bhatia D, Myerson MS, Curtis MJ, et al. Anatomical restraints to dislocation of the second metatarsophalangeal joint and assessment of a repair technique. J Bone Joint Surg Am 1994;76(9):1371–5.

19. Kaz AJ, Coughlin MJ. Crossover second toe: demographics, etiology, and radiographic assessment. Foot Ankle Int 2007;28(12):1223–37.

20. Borne J, Bordet B, Fantino O, et al. Plantar plate and second ray syndrome: normal and pathological US imaging features and proposed US classification. J Radiol 2010;91(5 Pt 1):543–8 [in French].

21. Bouche RT, Heit EJ. Combined plantar plate and hammertoe repair with flexor digitorum longus tendon transfer for chronic, severe sagittal plane instability of the lesser metatarsophalangeal joints: preliminary observations. J Foot Ankle Surg 2008; 47(2):125–37.

22. Brunet JA, Tubin S. Traumatic dislocations of the lesser toes. Foot Ankle Int 1997;18(7):406–11.

23. Mann RA, Mizel MS. Monarticular nontraumatic synovitis of the metatarsophalangeal joint: a new diagnosis? Foot Ankle 1985;6(1):18–21.

24. Mann RA, Coughlin MJ. The rheumatoid foot: review of literature and method of treatment. Orthop Rev 1979;8:105–12.

25. Deland JT, Sung IH. The medial crosssover toe: a cadaveric dissection. Foot Ankle Int 2000;21(5): 375–8.

26. Yu GV, Judge MS, Hudson JR, et al. Predislocation syndrome. Progressive subluxation/dislocation of the lesser metatarsophalangeal joint. J Am Podiatric Med Assoc 2002;92(4):182–99.

27. Barg A, Courville XF, Nickisch F, et al. Role of collateral ligaments in metatarsophalangeal stability: a cadaver study. Foot Ankle Int 2012;33(10): 877–82.

28. Powless SH, Elze ME. Metatarsophalangeal joint capsule tears: an analysis by arthrography, a new classification system and surgical management. J foot Ankle Surg 2001;40(6):374–89.

29. Morton DJ. Metatarsus atavicus:the identification of a distinctive type of foot disorder. J Bone Joint Surg 1927;(9):531–44.

30. Fleischer AE, Klein EE, Ahmad M, et al. Association of abnormal metatarsal parabola with second metatarsophalangeal joint plantar plate pathology. Foot Ankle Int 2017;38(3):289–97.

31. Murphy JL. Isolated dorsal dislocation of the second metatarsophalangeal joint. Foot Ankle 1980; 1(1):30–2.

32. Rao JP, Banzon MT. Irreducible dislocation of the metatarsophalangeal joints of the foot. Clin orthopaedics Relat Res 1979;(145):224–6.

33. Klein EE, Weil L Jr, Weil LS Sr, et al. Clinical examination of plantar plate abnormality: a diagnostic perspective. Foot Ankle Int 2013;34(6):800–4.

34. Coughlin MJ, Pinsonneault T. Operative treatment of interdigital neuroma. A long-term follow-up study. J Bone Joint Surg Am 2001;83(9):1321–8.

35. Mulder JD. The causative mechanism in morton's metatarsalgia. J Bone Joint Surg Br 1951;33-B(1): 94–5.

36. Trepman E, Yeo SJ. Nonoperative treatment of metatarsophalangeal joint synovitis. Foot Ankle Int 1995;16(12):771–7.

37. Thompson FM, Hamilton WG. Problems of the second metatarsophalangeal joint. Orthopedics 1987; 10(1):83–9.

38. Klein EE, Weil L Jr, Weil LS, et al. The underlying osseous deformity in plantar plate tears: a radiographic analysis. Foot Ankle Spec 2013;6(2):108–18.

39. Blitz NM, Ford LA, Christensen JC. Second metatarsophalangeal joint arthrography: a cadaveric correlation study. J Foot Ankle Surg 2004;43(4): 231–40.

40. Yao L, Cracchiolo A, Farahani K, et al. Magnetic resonance imaging of plantar plate rupture. Foot Ankle Int 1996;17(1):33–6.

41. Sung W, Weil L Jr, Weil LS Sr, et al. Diagnosis of plantar plate injury by magnetic resonance imaging with reference to intraoperative findings. J Foot Ankle Surg 2012;51(5):570–4.

42. Klein EE, Weil L Jr, Weil LS, et al. Musculoskeletal ultrasound for preoperative imaging of the plantar plate: a prospective analysis. Foot Ankle Spec 2013; 6(3):196–200.

43. Klein EE, Weil L Jr, Weil LS, et al. Magnetic resonance imaging versus musculoskeletal ultrasound for identification and localization of plantar plate tears. Foot Ankle Spec 2012;5(6):359–65.

44. Haddad SL, Sabbagh RC, Resch S, et al. Results of flexor-to-extensor and extensor brevis tendon transfer for correction of the crossover second toe deformity. Foot Ankle Int 1999;20(12):781–8.

45. Gregg J, Silberstein M, Clark C, et al. Plantar plate repair and Weil osteotomy for metatarsophalangeal joint instability. Foot Ankle Surg 2007;13(3): 116–21.

46. Ford LA, Collins KB, Christensen JC. Stabilization of the subluxed second metatarsophalangeal joint: flexor tendon transfer versus primary repair of the plantar plate. J Foot Ankle Surg 1998;37(3):217–22.

47. Coughlin MJ. Common causes of pain in the forefoot in adults. J Bone Joint Surg Br 2000;82(6): 781–90.

48. Myerson MS, Jung HG. The role of toe flexor-to-extensor transfer in correcting metatarsophalangeal

joint instability of the second toe. Foot Ankle Int 2005;26(9):675–9.

49. Phisitkul P, Hosuru Siddappa V, Sittapairoj T, et al. Cadaveric evaluation of dorsal intermetatarsal approach for plantar plate and lateral collateral ligament repair of the lesser metatarsophalangeal joints. Foot Ankle Int 2017;8(7):791–6.

50. Jastifer JR, Coughlin MJ. Exposure via sequential release of the metatarsophalangeal joint for plantar plate repair through a dorsal approach without an intraarticular osteotomy. Foot Ankle Int 2015;36(3): 335–8.

51. Finney FT, Lee S, Scott J, et al. Biomechanical evaluation of suture configurations in lesser toe plantar plate repairs. Foot Ankle Int 2018;39(7): 836–42.

52. Gallentine JW, DeOrio JK. Removal of the second toe for severe hammertoe deformity in elderly patients. Foot Ankle Int 2005;26(5):353–8.

53. Sarrafian SK, Topouzian LK. Anatomy and physiology of the extensor apparatus of the toes. J Bone Joint Surg Am 1969;51(4):669–79.

54. Prissel MA, Hyer CF, Donovan JK, et al. Plantar plate repair using a direct plantar approach: an outcomes analysis. J Foot Ankle Surg 2017;56(3):434–9.

55. Flint WW, Macias DM, Jastifer JR, et al. Plantar plate repair for lesser metatarsophalangeal joint instability. Foot Ankle Int 2017;38(3):234–42.

56. Nery C, Coughlin MJ, Baumfeld D, et al. Prospective evaluation of protocol for surgical treatment of lesser MTP joint plantar plate tears. Foot Ankle Int 2014;35(9):876–85.

57. Sung W. Technique using interference fixation repair for plantar plate ligament disruption of lesser metatarsophalangeal joints. J foot Ankle Surg 2015; 54(3):508–12.

58. Cook J, Cook E, Hansen D, et al. One-year outcome study of anatomic reconstruction of lesser metatarsophalangeal joints. Foot Ankle Spec 2020; 13(4):286–96.

59. Jastifer J, Doty J, Claassen L. Current concepts in the treatment of metatarsophalangeal joint instability of the lesser toes: Review, surgical technique, and early outcomes. Fuß Sprunggelenk 2017;15.

Moving?

Make sure your subscription moves with you!

To notify us of your new address, find your **Clinics Account Number** (located on your mailing label above your name), and contact customer service at:

Email: journalscustomerservice-usa@elsevier.com

800-654-2452 (subscribers in the U.S. & Canada)
314-447-8871 (subscribers outside of the U.S. & Canada)

Fax number: 314-447-8029

Elsevier Health Sciences Division
Subscription Customer Service
3251 Riverport Lane
Maryland Heights, MO 63043

Printed and bound by CPI Group (UK) Ltd, Croydon, CR0 4YY

08/05/2025

01864723-0013